Yoga: The Science of the Soul

Also by OSHO

Art of Tea
Autobiography of a Spiritually Incorrect Mystic
Awareness
The Book of Secrets
Courage
Creativity
India My Love: A Spiritual Journey
Intimacy
Intuition
Love, Freedom and Aloneness
Maturity
Meditation
Osho on Zen
Osho Transformation Tarot
Osho Zen Tarot
Sex Matters

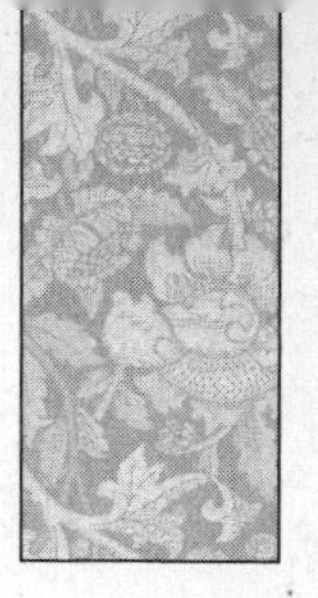

Yoga: The Science of the Soul

Osho

A Stream of Consciousness Reader

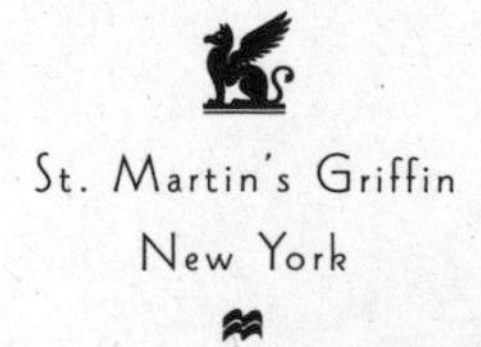

St. Martin's Griffin
New York

 Printed in the United States of America. For information, address St. Martin's Press, 175 Fifth Avenue, New York, N.Y. 10010.

www.stmartins.com

The material in this book has been selected from a series of one hundred talks given by Osho under the title "Yoga: The Alpha and the Omega."

Library of Congress Cataloging-in-Publication Data

Osho, 1931–1990.
Yoga : the science of the soul / Osho.—1st ed.
p. cm.
ISBN 0-312-30614-8
1. Spiritual life. 2. Yoga. I. Title.

BP605.R34 Y64 2002
299'.93—dc21

2002068398

10 9

CONTENTS

Yoga: The Science of the Soul

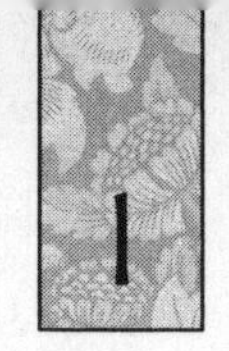

NOW THE DISCIPLINE OF YOGA

Now the discipline of yoga.
Yoga is the cessation of mind.
Then the witness is established in itself.
In the other states there is identification with the modifications of the mind.

We live in a deep illusion—the illusion of hope, of future, of tomorrow. As man is, man cannot exist without self-deceptions. Nietzsche says somewhere that man cannot live with the true: He needs dreams, he needs illusions, he needs lies in order to exist. And Nietzsche is right. As man is, he cannot exist with the truth. This has to be understood very deeply because without understanding it, there can be no entry into the inquiry that is called yoga.

The mind has to be understood deeply—the mind that needs lies, the mind that needs illusions, the mind that cannot exist with the real, the mind that needs dreams. You are not dreaming only during the night. Even while awake, you are dreaming continuously. You may be looking at me, you may be listening to me, but a dream current goes on within you. Continuously, the mind is creating dreams, images, fantasies.

Now scientists say that a person can live without sleep but not without dreams. In the old days it was understood that sleep is a necessity, but modern research now says sleep is not really a necessity. Sleep is needed only so that you can dream. The dream is the necessity. If you are allowed to sleep but not allowed to dream, you will not feel fresh and alive in the morning. You will feel tired, as if you have not been able to sleep at all.

During the night there are different periods—periods for deep sleep and periods for dreaming. There is a rhythm—just like day and night, there is a rhythm. In the beginning you fall into deep sleep for about forty or forty-five minutes. Then the dream phase comes in; then you dream. Then again dreamless sleep, then again dreaming. The whole night this goes on. If your sleep is disturbed while you are deeply asleep without dreaming, in the morning you will not feel that you have missed anything. But while you are dreaming, if your dream is disturbed, then in the morning you will feel completely tired and exhausted.

Now, this can be known from the outside—if someone is sleeping you can judge whether he is dreaming or asleep. If he is dreaming, his eyes will be moving constantly, as if he is watching something with closed eyes. When he is fast asleep, the eyes will not move; they will remain steady. So if your sleep is disturbed while your eyes are moving, in the morning you will feel tired. While your eyes are not moving, your sleep can be disturbed, and in the morning you will not feel anything is missing.

Many researchers have proved that the human mind feeds on dreams, that dreaming is a necessity, and that a dream is a total autodeception. And this is not only so in the night: While awake the same pattern also follows; even during the day you can notice it. Sometimes there will be dreams floating in the mind, sometimes there will be no dreams.

When there are dreams, you might be doing something, but you will be absent. Inside you are occupied. For example, you are here. If your mind is passing through a dream state, you will listen to me without listening at all because your mind will be occupied within. If you are not in a dreaming state, only then you can listen to me.

Day and night, the mind goes on moving from no dream to dream, then from dream to no dream again. This is an inner rhythm. Not only do we continuously dream, in life we also project hopes into the future.

The present is almost always a hell. You can endure it only because of the hopes that you have projected into the future. You can live today because of the tomorrow. You are hoping something is going to happen tomorrow, some doors to paradise will open tomorrow. They never open today. And when tomorrow comes, it will not come as a tomorrow, it will come as today—but by that time your mind has moved again. You go on moving ahead of yourself—this is what dreaming means. You are not one with the real, that which is nearby, that which is here and now; you are somewhere else, moving ahead, jumping ahead.

And that tomorrow, that future, you have named in so many ways. People call it "heaven," some people call it *moksha,* but it is always in the future. Somebody is thinking in terms of wealth—but that wealth is going to be in the future. Somebody is thinking in terms of paradise, and that paradise is going to be after you are dead—far away into the future.

You waste your present for that which is not. This is what dreaming means. You cannot be here and now; that seems to be arduous, to be just in the moment.

You can be in the past because that is again dreaming—memories, remembrance of things that are no more. Or you can be in the future, which is projection, which is again creating something out of the past. The future is nothing but the past projected again—more colorful, more beautiful, more pleasant, but it is the past refined.

You cannot think of anything other than the past. The future is nothing but the past projected again—and both are not! The present is—but you are never in the present. This is what dreaming means. And Nietzsche is right when he says that man cannot live with the truth. He needs lies, he lives through lies. Nietzsche says that we go on saying we want the truth, but no one wants it. Our so-called truths are nothing but lies, beautiful lies. No one is ready to see the naked reality.

This mind cannot enter on the path of yoga because yoga means a methodology to reveal the truth. Yoga is a method to come to a nondreaming mind. Yoga is the science to be in the here and now. Yoga means now you are ready not to move into the future. Yoga means you are ready now not to hope, not to jump ahead of your being. Yoga means to encounter the reality as it is.

If you are still hoping that you can gain something through your mind, yoga is not for you. A total frustration is needed, a revelation that this projecting mind is futile, that the mind that hopes is nonsense and leads nowhere.

So you can enter yoga, or the path of yoga, only when you are totally frustrated with your own mind as it is. If you are still hoping that you can gain something through your mind, yoga is not for you. A total frustration is needed, a revelation that this projecting mind is futile, that the mind that hopes is nonsense and leads nowhere. It simply closes your eyes; it intoxicates you. It never allows reality to be revealed to you. It protects you against reality. Your mind is a drug. It is against that which is. So unless you are totally frustrated with your mind, with your way of being, with the way you have existed up to now—if you can drop it unconditionally, then you can enter on the path.

So many become interested, but very few enter. Your interest may be just because of your mind. You may be hoping that now, through yoga, you may gain something. But the achieving motive is there: You might become perfect through yoga, you might reach the blissful state of perfect being. You might become one with the universal, you might achieve enlightenment—this may be why you are interested in yoga. If this is the cause of your interest, then there can be no meeting between you and the path that is yoga. Then you are totally against it, moving in a totally different dimension.

Yoga means that now there is no hope, now there is no future, now there are no desires. One is ready to know what *is.* One is not interested in what can be, what should be, what ought to be. One is not interested! One is interested only in that which is because only the real can free you. Only the reality can become liberation.

Total despair is needed. That despair is called *dukkha* by Buddha. If you are really in misery, don't hope because your hope will only prolong the misery. Your hope is a drug. It can help you to reach only death and nowhere else. All your hopes can lead you only to death—they *are* leading you.

Become totally hopeless—no future, no hope. It is difficult. It needs courage to face the real. But such a moment comes to everyone at some time or other. A moment comes to every human being when he feels total hopelessness. Absolute meaninglessness happens to him—when he becomes aware that whatever he is doing is useless, wherever he is going, he is going nowhere; all life is meaningless. Suddenly hope drops, future drops, and for the first time you are in tune with the present. For the first time you are face to face with reality. Unless this moment comes to you . . .

You can go on doing *asanas,* postures; that is not yoga. Yoga is an inward turning. It is a total about-face. When you are not moving into the future, not moving toward the past, then you start moving within yourself—because your being is here and now, it is not in the future. You are present here and now, you can enter this reality. But then the mind has to be here also. This moment is indicated by this sutra, this verse of Patanjali.

Yoga is an inward turning. It is a total about-face. When you are not moving into the future, not moving toward the past, then you start moving within yourself—because your being is here and now.

Before we talk about this first sutra, a few other things have to be understood.

First, yoga is not a religion—remember that. Yoga is not Hindu, it is not Mohammedan. Yoga is a pure science just like mathematics, physics, or chemistry. Physics is not Christian, physics is not Buddhist. Even if Christians have discovered the laws of physics, physics is not Christian. It is just accidental that Christians came to discover the laws of physics; physics is just a science. Yoga is a science—it is just an accident that Hindus discovered it. It is not Hindu; it is a pure mathematics of the inner being. So a Mohammedan can be a yogi, a Christian can be a yogi, a Jain or a Buddhist can be a yogi.

Yoga is pure science, and Patanjali is the greatest name as far as the world of yoga is concerned. This man is rare. There is no other name comparable to Patanjali. For the first time in the history of humanity, this man brought religion to the state of a science; he made religion a science, bare laws.

For yoga, no belief is needed. So-called religions need beliefs. There is no other difference between one religion and another; the difference is only of beliefs. A Mohammedan has certain beliefs, a Hindu certain others, a Christian certain others; the difference is of beliefs. Yoga has nothing as far as belief is concerned; yoga doesn't say to believe in anything. Yoga says, "Experience." Just like science says experiment, yoga says experience. Experiment and experience are the same; just their directions are different. Experiment is something you can do outside; experience is something you can do inside. Experience is an inside experiment.

Science says, "Don't believe; doubt as much as you can. But also, don't disbelieve because disbelief is again a sort of belief." You can believe in God, or you can believe in the concept of "no-God." You can say God exists, with a fanatical attitude, or you can say quite the reverse, that God does not exist—with the same fanaticism! Atheists, theists—all are believers, and belief is not the realm for science. Science means the experience of something, of that which is. No belief is needed.

> Yoga is existential, experiential, experimental. No belief is required, no faith is needed—only courage to experience.

So the second thing to remember is that yoga is existential, experiential, experimental. No belief is required, no faith is needed—only courage to experience. And that's what is lacking. You can believe easily because in belief you are not going to be transformed. Belief is something added to you, something superficial. Your being is not changed, you are not passing through some mutation. You may be a Hindu, and you can become Christian the next day. Simply, you change: You exchange the Gita for a Bible; you can exchange it for a Koran. But the man who was holding a Gita and is now holding the Bible remains the same. He has changed his beliefs.

Beliefs are like clothes. Nothing substantial is transformed; you remain the same. Dissect a Hindu, dissect a Mohammedan, and inside they are the same. The Hindu goes to a temple, and the Mohammedan hates the temple. The Mohammedan goes to the mosque, and the Hindu hates the mosque. But inside they are the same human beings.

Belief is easy because you are not required to really do anything—just a superficial dressing, a decoration, something that you can put aside at any moment you like. Yoga is not belief. That's why it is difficult, arduous, and sometimes it seems impossible. It is an existential approach. You will come to the truth not through belief but through your own experience, through your own realization. That means you will have to be totally changed. Your viewpoints, your way of life, your mind, your psyche has to be shattered completely as it is. Something new has to be created. Only with that "new" will you come in contact with the reality.

So yoga is both a death and a new life. As you are, you will have to die; and unless you die, the new cannot be born. The new is hidden in you. You are just a seed for it, and the seed must fall down and be absorbed by the earth. The seed must die; only then will the new arise out of you. Your death will become your new life. Yoga is both a death and a new birth. Unless you are ready to die, you cannot be reborn. So it is not a question of changing beliefs.

Yoga is not a philosophy. I say it is not a religion, and I say it is not a philosophy. It is not something you can think about. It is something you will have to *be;* thinking won't do. Thinking goes on in your head; it is not really deep into the roots of your being. It is not your totality. It is just a part, a functional part; it can be trained. And you can argue logically, you can think rationally, but your heart will remain the same. Your heart is your deepest center; your head is just a branch. You can be without the head, but you cannot be without the heart. Your head is not basic.

Yoga is concerned with your total being, with your roots. It is not philosophical. So with Patanjali we will not be thinking, speculating. With Patanjali we will be trying to know the ultimate laws of being—the laws of its transformation, the laws of how to die and how to be reborn again, the laws of a new order of being. That is why I call it a science.

Patanjali is rare. He is an enlightened person like Buddha, like Krishna, like Christ, like Mahavira, Mohammed, Zarathustra. But he is different in one way. Buddha, Krishna, Mahavira, Zarathustra, Mohammed—none of them has a scientific attitude. They are great founders of religions, they have changed the whole pattern of the human mind and its structure, but their approach is not scientific.

Patanjali is like an Einstein in the world of Buddhas. He is a phenomenon. He could have easily been a Nobel Prize winner like an Einstein or Bohr or Max Planck, a Heisenberg. He has the same attitude, the same rigorous, scientific approach. He is not a poet; Krishna is a poet. He is not a moralist; Mahavira is a moralist. He is basically a scientist thinking in terms of laws. And he has come to deduce absolute laws of the human being, the ultimate working structure of human mind and reality.

And if you follow Patanjali, you will come to know that he is as exact as any mathematical formula. Simply do what he says, and the result will happen. The result is bound to happen; it is just like two plus two, they become four. It is just like heating water up to the boiling point and it evaporates. No belief is needed; you simply do it, and you know. It is something to be done and known. That's why I say there is no comparison. On this earth, never has a man existed like Patanjali.

You can find poetry in Buddha's utterances—they are bound to be there. Many times while Buddha is expressing himself, he becomes poetic. The realm of ecstasy, the realm of ultimate knowing, is so beautiful, the temptation is so great to become poetic. The beauty is such, the benediction is such, the bliss is such that one starts talking in poetic language.

But Patanjali resists that. It is very difficult—no one has been able to resist. Jesus, Krishna, Buddha—they all become poetic. The splendor, the beauty—when it explodes within you, you will start dancing, you will start singing. In that state you are just like a lover who has fallen in love with the whole universe.

Patanjali resists that. He will not use poetry; he will not use even a single poetic symbol. He will not do anything with poetry; he will not talk in terms of beauty. He will talk in terms of mathematics. He will be exact, and he will give you maxims. Those maxims are just indications of what is to be done. He will not explode into ecstasy; he will not say things that cannot be said; he will not try the impossible. He will just put down the foundation, and if you

Patanjali will talk in terms of mathematics. He will be exact, and he will give you maxims. Those maxims are just indications of what is to be done.

follow the foundation, you will reach the peak that is beyond. He is a rigorous mathematician—remember this.

The first sutra:

Now the discipline of yoga.

Each and every word has to be understood because Patanjali will not use a single superfluous word.

Now the discipline of yoga.

First try to understand the word *now.* This "now" indicates toward the state of mind I was just talking to you about.

If you are disillusioned, if you are hopeless, if you have completely become aware of the futility of all desires, if you see your life as meaningless . . . If whatever you have been doing up to now has simply fallen dead, nothing remains in the future; you are in absolute despair—what Kierkegaard calls "anguish." . . . If you are in anguish, suffering, not knowing what to do, not knowing where to go, not knowing to whom to look, just on the verge of madness or suicide or death, and your whole pattern of life suddenly has become futile . . . If this moment has come, Patanjali says, *Now the discipline of yoga.* Only now can you understand the science of yoga, the discipline of yoga.

If that moment has not come, you can go on studying yoga, you can become a great scholar, but you will not be a yogi. You can write theses about it, you can give discourses on it, but you will not be a yogi. The moment has not come for you. Intellectually you can become interested. Through your mind you can be related to yoga. But yoga is nothing if it is not a discipline. Yoga is not a *shastra;* it is not a scripture. It is a discipline. It is something you have to *do.* It is not a curiosity; it is not philosophical speculation. It is deeper than that. It is a question of life and death.

If the moment has come where you feel that all directions have become confused, all roads have disappeared—the future is dark, and every desire has become bitter, and through every desire you have known only disappointment; all movement into hopes and dreams has ceased—*Now the discipline of yoga.*

This "now" may not have come. I can go on talking about yoga, but you will not listen. You can listen only if the moment is present in you.

Are you really dissatisfied? Everybody will say yes, but that dissatisfaction is not real. You are dissatisfied with this, you may be dissatisfied with that, but you are not totally dissatisfied. You are still hoping. You are dissatisfied because of your past hopes, but for the future you are still hoping. Your dissatisfaction is not total. You are still hankering for some satisfaction somewhere, for some gratification somewhere.

Sometimes you feel hopeless, but that hopelessness is not true. You feel hopeless because certain hopes have not been achieved, certain hopes have fallen. But *hoping* is still there; hoping has not fallen. You will still hope. You are dissatisfied with this hope, that hope, but you are not dissatisfied with hope as such. If you are disappointed with hope as such, then the moment has come—and you can enter yoga. Then this entry will not be entering into a mental, speculative phenomenon. This entry will be an entry into a discipline.

What is discipline? Discipline means creating an order within you. As you are, you are a chaos. As you are, you are totally disorderly. George Gurdjieff used to say—and Gurdjieff is in many ways like Patanjali; he was again trying to make the core of religion a science—Gurdjieff says that you are not one, you are a crowd. Not even when you say "I" is there any "I." There are many "I's" in you, many egos. In the morning, one "I," in the afternoon, another "I," in the evening, a third "I." But you never become aware of this mess because who will become aware of it? There is no center that can become aware.

To say that yoga is discipline means yoga wants to create a crystallized center in you. As you are, you are a crowd. And a crowd has many phenomena. One is that you cannot believe a crowd. Gurdjieff used to say that man cannot promise. Who will promise? You are not there! If you promise, who will fulfill the promise? Next morning the one who promised is no more.

People come to me, and they say, "Now I will take a vow; I promise to do this." I tell them. "Think twice before you promise something. Are you confident that the next moment the one who promised will be there?" You decide to get up early in the morning, starting tomorrow—at four o'clock. But at four o'clock somebody in you says, "Don't bother. It is so cold outside . . . and why are you in such a hurry? We can do it tomorrow." And you fall asleep again. When you get up, you repent, and you think, "This is not good. I should have done it." You decide again: "Tomorrow I will do it." And the same is going to happen tomorrow because at four in the morning the one who promised is no longer there; somebody else is in the chair. You are a Rotary Club! The chairman goes on changing; every member becomes a rotary chairman. Every moment someone else is the master.

Think twice before you promise something. Are you confident that the next moment the one who promised will be there?

Gurdjieff used to say, "This is the chief characteristic of

man, that he cannot promise." You cannot fulfill a promise. You go on giving promises, and you know well that you cannot fulfill them. It is because you are not one; you are a disorder, a chaos. Hence, Patanjali says, *Now the discipline of yoga.* If your life has become an absolute misery, if you have realized that whatsoever you do creates hell, then the moment has come.

This moment can change your dimension, your direction of being. Up until now you have lived as a chaos, a crowd. Yoga means that now you will have to be a harmony, you will have to become one. Crystallization is needed; centering is needed. And unless you attain a center, all that you do is useless; it is wasting life and time. A center is the first necessity, and only a person who has a center can be blissful. Everybody asks for blissfulness, but you cannot *ask* for it, you have to *earn* it! Everybody hankers for a blissful state of being, but only a center can be blissful. A crowd cannot be blissful, a crowd has no self. Who is going to be blissful?

Bliss means absolute silence, and silence is possible only when there is harmony—when all the discordant fragments have become one, when there is no crowd, but one. When you are alone in the house and nobody else is there, you will be blissful. Right now everybody else is in your house—*you* are not there. Only guests are there. The host is always absent—and only the host can be blissful.

This centering Patanjali calls discipline—*anushasanam.* The word *discipline* is beautiful. It comes from the same root as the word *disciple.* Discipline means the capacity to learn, the capacity to know. But you cannot know, you cannot learn, unless you have attained the capacity to *be.*

A man once came to Buddha, and he said—he must have been a social reformer, a revolutionary—he said to Buddha, "The world is in misery. I agree with you." But Buddha never said that the world is in misery. Buddha says *you* are the misery, not the world. Life is misery, not the world. Man is misery, not the world. Mind is misery, not the world. But that revolutionary said, "The world is in misery. I agree with you. Now, tell me, what can I do? I have a deep compassion, and I want to serve humanity."

Service must have been his motto. Buddha looked at him and remained silent. Buddha's disciple, Ananda, said, "This man seems to be sincere. Guide him. Why are you silent?" Then Buddha said to that revolutionary, "You want to serve the world, but where are you? I don't see anyone inside. I look in you, and there is no one. You don't have any center, and unless you are centered, whatsoever you do will create more mischief."

All of your social reformers, your revolutionaries, your leaders, they are the great mischief mongers. The world would be better if there were no leaders. But they cannot help themselves. They must do something because the world is in misery. And they are not centered, so whatever they do, they create more misery. Just compassion will not help, just service will not help. Compassion that flows through a centered being is something totally different. Compassion coming through a crowd is mischief. That compassion is poison.

Now the discipline of yoga.

Discipline means the capacity to be, the capacity to know, the capacity to learn. We must understand these three things.

The capacity to be—all the yoga postures are not really concerned with the body, they are concerned with the capacity to be. Patanjali says if you can sit silently without moving your body for a few hours, you are growing in the capacity to be. Why do you move? You cannot sit without moving even for a few seconds. Your body starts moving; somewhere you feel itching, the legs go dead, many things start happening—these are just excuses for you to move.

You are not a master. You cannot say to the body, "Now, for one hour I will not move." The body will revolt immediately! Immediately it will force you to move, to do something, and it will give reasons: "You have to move because an insect is biting you." You may not find the insect when you look. . . .

You are not a being, you are a trembling—a continuous, hectic activity. Patanjali's *asanas,* postures, are concerned not really with any kind of physiological training but an inner training of being. Just to be—without doing anything, without any movement, without any activity; just remain. That "remaining" will help centering. If you can remain in one posture, the body will become a servant; it will follow you. And the more the body follows you, the greater being you will have within you, a stronger being within you.

Patanjali's postures are concerned not really with any kind of physiological training but an inner training of being. Just to be—without doing anything, without any movement.

And remember, if the body is not moving, your mind cannot move because mind and body are not two things. They are two poles of one phenomenon. You are not body and mind, you are body-mind. Your personality is psychosomatic—body-mind both. The mind is the subtlest part of the body. Or you can say the reverse, that body is the grossest part of the mind. So whatever happens in the body happens in the mind, and vice versa: Whatever happens in the mind happens in the body. If the body is nonmoving and you can attain a posture—if you can say to the body, "Keep quiet"—the mind will remain silent. Really, the mind starts moving and tries to move the body because if the body moves, then the mind can move. In a nonmoving body the mind cannot move; it needs a moving body.

If the body is nonmoving, the mind is nonmoving, you are centered. This nonmoving posture is not just a physiological training. It is to create a situation in which centering can happen, in which you can become disciplined. When you *are,* when you have become centered, when you know what it means to be, then you can learn. Because then you will be humble, then you can surrender. Then no false ego will cling to you because once centered, you know all egos are false. Then you can bow down. Then a disciple is born.

A disciple means a seeker who is not a crowd, who is trying to be centered and crystallized, at least trying, making efforts, sincere efforts, to become individual, to feel his being, to become his own master. All discipline of yoga is an effort to make you a master of yourself. As you are, you are just a slave of many, many desires. Many, many masters are there, and you are just a slave—and pulled in many directions.

Now the discipline of yoga.

Yoga is discipline. It is an effort on your part to change yourself.

Many other things have to be understood. Yoga is not a therapy. In the West many psychological therapies are prevalent now, and many western psychologists think that yoga is also a therapy. It is not! It is a discipline. And what is the difference? This is the difference: A therapy is needed if you are ill, a therapy is needed if you are diseased, a therapy is needed if you are pathological. A discipline is needed even when you are healthy. Really, a discipline can help *only* when you are healthy. It is not for pathological cases. Yoga is for those who are completely healthy as far as medical science is concerned; normal. They are not schizophrenic, they are not mad, they are not neurotic. They are normal people, healthy people with no particular pathology. Still, they become aware that whatever is called "normality" is futile, whatever is called "health" is of no use. Something more is needed, something greater is needed; something more whole is needed.

Therapies are for ill people. Therapies can help you to come to yoga, but yoga is not a therapy. Yoga is for a higher order of health, a different order of health—a different type of being and wholeness. Therapy can, at the most, make you adjusted. Freud says we cannot do more. We can make you an adjusted, normal member of the society—but if the society itself is pathological, then? And it is! The society itself is ill. A therapy can make you normal in the sense that you are adjusted to the society, but the society itself is ill.

So sometimes it happens that in an ill society a healthy person is thought to be ill. A Jesus is thought to be ill, and every effort is done to make him adjusted. And when it is found that he is a hopeless case, then he is crucified. When it is found that nothing can be done, this man is incurable, then he is crucified. The society is itself ill because society is nothing but your collective. If all the members are ill, the society is ill—and every member has to be adjusted to it.

Yoga is not therapy. Yoga is not trying in any way to make you adjusted to the society. If you want to define yoga in terms of adjustment, then it is not an adjustment with the society but an adjustment with existence itself. It is an adjustment with the whole.

So it might happen that a perfect yogi could appear mad to

you. He may look out of his senses, out of his mind, because now he is in touch with a higher mind, a higher order of things. He is in touch with the universal mind. It has always happened so: A Buddha, a Jesus, a Krishna, they always look somehow eccentric. They don't belong to us; they seem to be outsiders.

> If you want to define yoga in terms of adjustment, then it is not an adjustment with the society but an adjustment with existence itself. It is an adjustment with the whole.

That's why we call them *avatars,* outsiders. It is as if they have come from some other planet; they don't belong to us. They may be higher, they may be good, they may be divine, but they don't belong to us. They come from somewhere else. They are not part and parcel of humankind.

The feeling has persisted that they are outsiders—they are not. They are the real insiders because they have touched the innermost core of existence. But to us they appear to be outsiders.

Now the discipline of yoga.

If your mind has come to realize that whatsoever you have been doing up to now was just senseless, it was a nightmare at the worst or a beautiful dream at the best, then the path of discipline opens before you. What is that path?

The basic definition is:

Yoga is the cessation of mind.

I said that Patanjali is just mathematical. In a single sentence—"Now the discipline of yoga"—he is finished with you.

This is the only sentence that has been used for you. Now he takes it for granted that you are interested in yoga not as a hope but as a discipline, as a transformation right here and now. He proceeds to define it:

Yoga is the cessation of mind.

This is the best definition of yoga. Yoga has been defined in many ways; there are many definitions. Some say yoga is the meeting of the mind with the whole; hence it is called "yoga"—*yoga* means meeting, joining together. Some say that yoga means dropping the ego: Ego is the barrier; the moment you drop the ego you are joined to the whole. You were already joined, only because of the ego it appeared that you were disjoined. And there are many other definitions, but Patanjali's is the most scientific. He says, *Yoga is the cessation of mind.*

Yoga is the state of "no-mind." The word *mind* covers all—your egos, your desires, your hopes, your philosophies, your religions, your scriptures. "Mind" covers all. Whatsoever you can think is mind. All that is known, all that can be known, all that is knowable, is within mind. Cessation of the mind means cessation of the known, cessation of the knowable. It is a jump into the unknown.

When there is no mind, you are in the unknown. Yoga is a jump into the unknown. Or, it will be better to say, the unknowable.

What is the mind? What is the mind doing there? What is it? Ordinarily we think that mind is something substantial there, inside the head. Patanjali doesn't agree—and no one who has ever known the inside of the mind will agree. Modern science also doesn't agree. Mind is not something substantial inside the head. Mind is just a function, just an activity.

You walk, and I say, "You are walking." What is walking? If you stop, where is walking? If you sit down, where has the walking gone? Walking is nothing substantial, it is an activity. So while you are sitting, no one can ask you, "Where have you put your walking? Just now you were walking, so where has the walking gone?" You will laugh. You will say, "Walking is not something substantial; it is just an activity. I can walk again. I can walk, and I can stop. It is an activity."

Mind is also an activity, but because of the word *mind,* it appears as if something substantial is there. It is better to call it "minding"—just like "walking." Mind means "minding"; mind means thinking. It is an activity.

I have quoted Bodhidharma many times:

> He traveled to China, and the emperor of China went to see him. The emperor said, "My mind is very uneasy, very disturbed. You are a great sage, and I have been waiting for you. Tell me what I should do to put my mind at peace."
>
> Bodhidharma replied, "You don't do anything. First you bring your mind to me."
>
> The emperor could not follow. He asked, "What do you mean?"
>
> Bodhidharma said, "Come in the morning at four o'clock when nobody is around. Come alone, and remember to bring your mind with you."
>
> The emperor couldn't sleep the whole night. Many times he cancelled the whole idea: "This man seems to be mad. What does he mean, 'Come with your mind; don't forget'?" But Bodhidarma was so enchanting, so charismatic, that the emperor couldn't cancel the appointment. As if a magnet

was pulling him, at four o'clock he jumped out of bed and said, "Whatever happens, I must go. This man may have something; his eyes say that he has something. Looks a little crazy, but still I must go and see what can happen."

So he went, and Bodhidharma was sitting there with his big staff. He said, "So you have come? Where is your mind? Have you brought it or not?"

The emperor replied, "You talk nonsense. When I am here, my mind is here, and it is not something that I can forget somewhere. It is in me."

So Bodhidharma said, "OK. So the first thing is decided—that the mind is within you."

The emperor said, "OK, the mind is within me."

Bodhidharma then said, "Now close your eyes and find out where it is. And if you can find out where it is, immediately indicate to me. I will put it at peace."

So the emperor closed his eyes, tried and tried, looked and looked. The more he looked, the more he became aware that there is no mind, that mind is an activity. It is not some *thing* that you can pinpoint. But the moment he realized that it is not some thing, then the absurdity of his quest was exposed to him. If the mind is not some thing, nothing can be done about it. If it is an activity, then don't do the activity; that's all. If it is like walking, don't walk.

The emperor opened his eyes. He bowed down to Bodhidharma and said, "There is no mind to be found."

Bodhidharma said, "Then I have put it at peace. And whenever you feel that you are uneasy, just look within, where that uneasiness is."

The very look is antimind because a look is not a "thinking." And if you look intensely, your whole energy becomes a look—the same energy that was movement and thinking before.

Yoga is the cessation of mind.

This is Patanjali's definition. When there is no mind, you are in yoga; when there is mind, you are not in yoga. So you may do all the postures, but if the mind goes on functioning, if you go on thinking, you are not in yoga.

Yoga is the state of no-mind. If you can be without the mind without doing any posture, you have become a perfect yogi. It has happened to many without doing any postures, and it has not happened to many who have been doing postures for many lives. Because the basic thing to be understood is this: When the activity of thinking is *not* there, *you* are there. When the activity of the mind is not there, when thoughts have disappeared—they are just like clouds—when they have disappeared, your being, just like the sky, is uncovered. It is always there, only it is covered with the clouds, covered with thoughts.

Yoga is the cessation of mind.

In the West now there is much appeal in Zen—a Japanese method of yoga. The word *zen* comes from *dhyana*. Bodhidharma introduced this word *dhyana* in China. In China the word *dhyana* became *jhan* and then *chan*, and then the word traveled to Japan and became *zen*. The root is *dhyana*, which means no-mind. So the whole training of Zen in Japan is of nothing but how to stop "minding," how to be a no-mind, how to be simply without thinking.

Try it! When I say try it, it will look contradictory . . . because there is no other way to say it. Because if you try, the very trying, the effort, is coming from the mind. You can sit in a posture, and you can try some *japa*—chanting, a mantra—or you can just try to sit silently, not to think. But then *not* to think becomes a thinking. You go on saying, "I am not to think . . . don't think . . . stop thinking." But this is all thinking.

Try to understand. When Patanjali talks about no-mind, cessation of mind, he means *complete cessation.* He will not allow you to create *japa*—"Ram-Ram-Ram." He will say that this is not cessation; you are using the mind. He will say, "Simply stop!"

But you will ask, "How? How to simply stop?" The mind continues. Even if you sit, the mind continues. Even if you don't do, it goes on doing.

Patanjali says, "Just look." Let mind go, let mind do whatsoever it is doing. You just look. You don't interfere. You just be a witness, you just be an onlooker, not concerned, as if the mind doesn't belong to you. As if it is not your business, not your concern. Don't be concerned! Just look, and let the mind flow. It is flowing because of past momentum, because you have always helped it to flow. The activity has taken on its own momentum, so it is flowing. You just don't cooperate. Look, and let the mind flow. For many, many lives, millions of lives maybe, you have cooperated with it. You have helped it, you have given your energy to it. The river will flow for a while. If you don't cooperate, if you just look unconcerned—Buddha's word is "indifference," *upeksha,* looking without any concern, just looking, not doing anything in any way—the mind will flow for a while, and it will stop by itself. When the momentum is lost, when the energy has flowed, the mind will stop.

When the mind stops, you are in yoga. You have attained the discipline. This is the definition:

Yoga is the cessation of mind.
Then the witness is established in itself.

When the mind ceases, the witness is established in itself. When you can simply look without being identified with the mind. Without judging, without appreciating or condemning, without choosing—you simply look, and the mind flows—a time comes when, by itself, of itself, the mind stops.

When there is no mind, you are established in your witnessing. Then you have become a witness—just a seer, *a drashta,* a *sakchhi.* Then you are not a doer. Then you are not a thinker. Then you are simply pure being, the purest of being. Then the witness is established in itself.

In the other states there is identification with the modifications of the mind.

Except witnessing, in all states you are identified with the mind. You become one with the flow of thoughts, you become one with the clouds—sometimes with the white cloud, sometimes with the black cloud, sometimes with a rain-filled cloud, sometimes with a vacant, empty cloud. But whatsoever the case, you become one with the thought, you become one with the cloud, and you miss your purity of sky, the purity of space. You become clouded, and this clouding happens because you get identified, you become one with the clouds.

A thought comes. You are hungry. And the thought flashes in the mind. The thought is simply that there is hunger, that the stomach is feeling hunger. Immediately you get identified; you say, "I am hungry." The mind was just filled with a thought that hunger is there, but you have become identified, and you say, "I am hungry." This is the identification.

Buddha also feels hunger, Patanjali also feels hunger, but

Patanjali will never say, "I am hungry." He will say, "The body is hungry." He will say, "My stomach is feeling hungry." He will say, "There is hunger. I am a witness. I have come to witness this thought, which has been flashed by the belly in the brain, saying 'I am hungry.' " The belly is hungry; Patanjali will remain a witness. You become identified; you become one with the thought.

Then the witness is established in itself.
In the other states there is identification with the modifications of the mind.

This is the definition:

Yoga is the cessation of mind.

When mind ceases, you are established in your witnessing self. In other states there are identifications, and all identifications constitute the world. If you are in the identifications, you are in the world, in the misery. If you have transcended the identifications, you are liberated. You have become a *siddha;* you are in *nirvana.* You have transcended this world of misery and entered the world of bliss.

And that world is here and now—right now, this very moment! You need not wait even a single moment for it. Just become a witness of the mind, and you have entered. Get identified with the mind, and you have missed. This is the basic definition.

Remember everything because later on, in other sutras, we will enter the details of what is to be done, how it is to be done—but always keep in mind that this is the foundation.

One has to achieve a state of no-mind. That is the goal.

2

THE FIVE MODIFICATIONS OF THE MIND

The modifications of the mind are five. They can be either a source of anguish or of nonanguish.
They are right knowledge, wrong knowledge, imagination, sleep, and memory.

MIND can be either the source of bondage or the source of freedom. Mind becomes the gate for this world, the entry; it can also become the exit. Mind leads you to hell, and mind can also lead you to heaven; it depends on how the mind is used.

Right use of the mind becomes meditation; wrong use of the mind becomes madness. Mind is there in everyone. The possibility of darkness and light are both implied in it. Mind itself is neither the enemy nor the friend. You can make it a friend, you can make it an enemy—it depends on you, on the one who is hidden behind the mind. If you can make the mind your instrument, your servant, the mind becomes the passage through which you can reach the ultimate. If you become the servant and the mind is allowed to be the master, then this mind that has become master will lead you to ultimate anguish and darkness.

All the techniques, all the methods, all the paths of yoga are really concerned deeply with only one problem: how to use the mind. Rightly used, mind comes to a point where it becomes no-mind. Wrongly used, mind comes to a point where it is just a chaos, many voices antagonistic to each other, contradictory, confusing, insane.

The madman in the madhouse and Buddha under his bodhi tree—both have used the mind. Both have passed through the mind. Buddha has come to a point where the mind disappears. Rightly used, it goes on disappearing, and a moment comes when it is not. The madman has also used the mind. Wrongly used, the mind becomes divided. Wrongly used, mind becomes many; wrongly used, it becomes a multitude, and finally the mad mind is there, and you are absolutely absent.

Buddha's mind has disappeared—and Buddha is present in his totality. A madman's mind has become total—and he himself has disappeared completely. These are the two poles, you and your mind. If they exist together, then you will be in misery. Either you will have to disappear or the mind will have to disappear. If the mind disappears, then you achieve truth. If you disappear, you achieve insanity. And this is the struggle: Who is going to disappear? Are you going to disappear or the mind? This is the conflict, the root of all struggle.

These sutras of Patanjali will lead you step by step toward this understanding of the mind: what it is, what modes it takes, what types of modifications come into it, how you can use it and go beyond it. And remember, you have nothing else right now—only the mind. You have to use it. If you use it wrongly, you will go on falling into more and more misery.

Patanjali will lead you step by step toward this understanding of the mind: what it is, what modes it takes, what types of modifications come into it, how you can use it and go beyond it.

You *are* in misery. That is

because for many lives you have used your mind wrongly, and the mind has become the master. You are just a slave, a shadow following the mind. You cannot say to the mind, "Stop." You cannot order your own mind; your mind goes on ordering you, and you have to follow it. Your being has become a shadow and a slave, an instrument in the hands of the mind.

Mind is nothing but an instrument, just like your hands or your feet. You order your feet, your legs, and they move. When you say "stop," they stop. You are the master. If I want to move my hand, I move it. If I don't want to move my hand, I don't move it. The hand cannot say to me, "Now I want to be moved." The hand cannot say to me, "Now I will move no matter what you do. I am not going to listen to you." If my hand starts moving in spite of me, then it will be a chaos in the body.

That's what has happened in the mind. You don't want to think, and the mind goes on thinking. You want to sleep. You are lying down on your bed, turning from side to side; you want to go to sleep, and the mind continues, the mind says, "No, I am going to think about something." You go on saying "stop," and it never listens to you, and you cannot do anything.

Mind is just an instrument, but you have given it too much power. It has become dictatorial, and it will struggle hard if you try to put it in its right place.

Buddha also uses the mind, but his mind is just like your legs. People go on coming to me, and they ask, "What happens to the mind of an enlightened one? Does it simply disappear? He cannot use it?"

It disappears as a master; it remains as a servant. It remains as a passive instrument. When Buddha wants to use the mind, he can use it. When Buddha speaks to you, he will have to use it because there is no possibility of speech without the mind. The mind has to be used. If you go to Buddha and he recognizes you, he knows that you have come before, he is using the mind. Without mind there can be no recognition; without mind there is no memory. But he *uses* the mind, remember—this is the distinction—and you are *being used by* the mind. Whenever Buddha wants to use the mind, he uses it. Whenever he doesn't want to use it, he doesn't use it. It is a passive instrument; it has no hold on him.

So Buddha remains like a mirror. If you come before the mirror, the mirror reflects you. When you have moved away, the reflection has gone, and the mirror is vacant. You are not like a mirror. You see somebody . . . the man has gone, but the thinking continues, the reflection continues. You go on thinking about him. And even if you want to stop, the mind won't listen.

Mastery of the mind is yoga. And when Patanjali talks about "cessation of the mind," this is what he means: It ceases as a master; mind ceases as a master. Then it is not active, then it is a passive instrument. You order, it works; you don't order, it remains still. It is just waiting. It cannot assert by itself. The assertion is lost; the violence is lost. It will not try to control you. Now just the reverse is the case.

How to become masters? How to put mind in its place, where you can use it—where, if you don't want to use it, you can put it aside and remain silent?

So the whole mechanism of the mind will have to be understood.

Now we should enter the sutra.

First:

The modifications of the mind are five. They can be either a source of anguish or of nonanguish.

The first thing to be understood is that mind is not something different from the body. Remember: Mind is part of the body. It is the body, but deeply subtle—a state of the body but very delicate, very refined. You cannot catch hold of it, but through the body you can influence it. If you take a drug, if you take LSD or marijuana or alcohol or something else, suddenly the mind is affected. The drug goes into the body, not into the mind, but the mind is affected. Mind is the subtlest part of the body.

The reverse is also true. Influence the mind, and the body is affected. That happens in hypnosis. A person who cannot walk, who says that he is paralyzed, can sometimes walk under hypnosis or you don't have any paralysis, but if under hypnosis you are told, "Now your body is paralyzed, and you cannot walk," you will not be able to walk. Sometimes paralyzed man can walk under hypnosis. What is happening? Hypnosis goes into the mind, the suggestion goes into the mind. Then the body follows.

That's the first thing to be understood: Mind and body are not two. This is one of the deepest discoveries of Patanjali. Now modern science recognizes it; it is very recent in the West. Now they say that to talk as if there is a dichotomy between body and mind is not right. Now they say it is a "psychosoma," it is mind-body. These two terms are just two functions of one phenomenon. One pole is mind, another pole is body, so you can work from either and change the other.

The body has five organs of activity—five *indriyas,* five instruments of activity. The mind has five modifications, five modes of function. Mind and body are one. The body is divided into five functions, and the mind is also divided into five functions. We will go into each function in detail.

The second part of this sutra is:

They can be either a source of anguish or of nonanguish.

These five modifications of the mind, this totality of the mind can lead you into deep anguish, what Buddha calls, *dukkha,* misery. Or, if you rightly use this mind and its functioning, it can lead you into nonmisery.

It can lead you at the most into nonmisery. That word *nonmisery* is very significant. Patanjali doesn't say that it will lead you into *ananda,* into bliss, no. The mind can lead you into misery if you wrongly use it, if you become a slave to it. If you become the master, the mind can lead you into nonmisery—not into bliss because bliss is your nature; the mind cannot lead you to it. But if you are in nonmisery, the inner bliss starts flowing.

Bliss is your intrinsic nature. It is nothing to be achieved and earned; it is nothing to be reached somewhere. You are born with it.

The bliss is always there inside; it is your intrinsic nature. It is nothing to be achieved and earned; it is nothing to be reached somewhere. You are born with it. You have it already; it is already the case. That's why Patanjali doesn't say that the mind can lead you into misery or can lead you into bliss. No, he is very scientific, very accurate. He will not use even a single word that can give you any untrue information. He simply says either misery or nonmisery.

Buddha also says this many times, whenever seekers come to him—seekers are after bliss, so they will ask Buddha, "How can we reach the ultimate bliss?" He will say, "I don't know. I can show you the path that leads to nonmisery, just the absence of misery. I don't say anything about the positive bliss, only the negative. I can show you how to move into the world of nonmisery."

That's all that methods can do. Once you are in the state of nonmisery, the inner bliss starts flowing. But that doesn't come from the mind, that comes from your inner being. So mind has nothing to do with it; mind cannot create it. If mind is in misery, then mind becomes a hindrance. If mind is in nonmisery, then mind becomes an opening. But it is not creative; it is not doing anything to create blissfulness. You open the windows, and the rays of the sun enter. By opening the windows, you are not creating the sun. The sun was already there. If it were not there, then just by opening the windows, the rays wouldn't enter. Your window can become a hindrance—the sunrays may be outside and the window is closed. The window can hinder or it can give way. It can become a passage, but it cannot be creative. It cannot create the rays; the rays are already there.

Your mind, if it is in misery, becomes closed. Remember, one of the characteristics of misery is closedness. Whenever you are in misery, you become closed. Observe: Whenever you feel some anguish, you are closed to the world. Even to your dearest friend you are closed. Even to your wife, your children, your beloved you are closed when you are in misery because misery because misery shrinks you inside. You shrink; from everywhere you have closed your doors.

That's why in misery, people start thinking of suicide. Suicide means total closure—no possibility of any communication, no possibility of any door. Even a closed door is dangerous. Someone can open it, so destroy the door; destroy all possibilities. Suicide means, "Now I am going to destroy all possibility of any opening. Now I am closing myself totally."

Whenever you are in misery, you start thinking of suicide. Whenever you are happy, you cannot think of suicide; you cannot imagine. You cannot even imagine why people commit suicide—life is such joy, life is such a deep music, why would people destroy life? It appears impossible.

Why, when you are happy, does it looks impossible? Because you are open; life is flowing in you. When you are happy, you have a bigger soul, you have expansion. When you are unhappy, you have a smaller soul, shrunken.

When someone is unhappy, touch him, take his hand into your hand—you will feel that his hand is dead. Nothing is flowing through it—no love, no warmth. It is just cold, as if it belonged to a corpse. When someone is happy, touch his hand—there is communication, energy is flowing. His hand is not just dead, his hand has become a bridge. Through his hand something comes to you, communicates, relates. Warmth flows. He reaches toward you, he makes every effort to flow into you, and he allows you also to flow within him.

When two persons are happy, they become one. That's why in love, oneness happens, and lovers start feeling that they are not two. They are two, but they start feeling they are not two because in love they are so happy that a melting happens. They melt into each other; they flow into each other. Boundaries dissolve, definitions are blurred, and they don't know who is who. In that moment they become one.

When you are happy, you can flow into others, and you can allow others to flow into you. This is what celebration means.

When you are happy, you can flow into others, and you can allow others to flow into you. This is what celebration means.

When you allow everybody to flow in and you flow into everybody, you are celebrating life. And celebration is the greatest prayer, the highest peak of meditation.

In misery you start thinking of committing suicide; in misery you start thinking of destruction. In misery you are on the opposite pole of celebration. You blame, you cannot celebrate. You have a grudge against everything. Everything is wrong, and you are negative, and you cannot flow, and you cannot relate, and you cannot allow anybody to flow into you. You have become an island, completely closed. This is a living death. Life is only when you are open and flowing, when you are unafraid, fearless, open, vulnerable, celebrating.

Patanjali says that the mind can do two things. It can create misery or nonmisery. You can use it in such a way that you can become miserable—and you have used it that way, you are past masters of it. There is no need to talk much about it; you know it already. You know the art of how to create misery. You may not be aware, but that is what you are doing continuously. Whatever you touch becomes a source of misery—and I repeat: whatever!

I see poor men. They are miserable, obviously. They are poor; the basic needs of life are not fulfilled. But then I see rich men, and they are also miserable. And these rich men think that wealth leads nowhere. That is not right. Wealth can lead to celebration, but you don't have the mind to celebrate. So if you are poor, you are miserable, and if you become rich, you are more miserable. The moment you touch the riches, you have destroyed them.

You have heard the Greek story of King Midas? Whatever he would touch, it turned into gold. You touch gold, and immediately it becomes mud. It is turned into dust, and then you think that there is nothing in this world, that even riches are useless.

They are not! But your mind cannot celebrate, your mind cannot participate in any nonmisery. If you are invited into heaven, you will not find heaven there; you will create a hell. As you are now, wherever you go, you will take your hell with you.

There is one Arabic proverb that says hell and heaven are not geographical places, they are attitudes. And no one enters heaven or hell; everybody enters *with* heaven or hell. Wherever you go, you carry your projection of hell or heaven with you. You have a projector inside—immediately you project.

Mind cannot give you bliss; no one can give it to you. It is hidden in you, and when mind is in a nonmiserable state, that bliss starts flowing. It is not coming from the mind, it is coming from beyond.

But Patanjali is careful. He says misery or "nonmisery"—positive misery or negative misery—but not "bliss." Mind cannot give you bliss; no one can give it to you. It is hidden in you, and when mind is in a nonmiserable state, that bliss starts flowing. It is not coming from the mind, it is coming from beyond. That's why Patanjali says the mind can be either a source of anguish or of nonanguish.

The modifications of the mind are five.
They are right knowledge, wrong knowledge, imagination, sleep, and memory.

The first modification of the mind is *praman*, right knowledge. The Sanskrit word *praman* is very deep and really cannot be translated. "Right knowledge" is just a shadow, not the exact meaning, because there is no word that can translate *praman. Praman* comes from the root *prama.* Many things have to be understood about it.

Patanjali says that the mind has a capacity. If that capacity is directed rightly, then whatsoever is known is true; it is self-evidently true. We are not aware of it because we have never used it; that faculty has remained unused. It is just as if the room is dark, you come into it, and you have a flashlight, but you are not using it—so the room remains dark. You go on stumbling against this table, over that chair—and you have a light! But the light has to be put on. Once you put the flashlight on, immediately the darkness disappears. Wherever the light is focused, you know, you can see. That spot at least becomes evident, self-evidently clear.

Mind has a capacity of *praman,* of right knowledge, of wisdom. Once you know how to switch it on, then wherever you move that light, only right knowledge is revealed. Without knowing how to turn on the light, whatever you know will be wrong.

Mind also has the capacity of wrong knowledge. In Sanskrit that wrong knowledge is called *viparyaya*—false, *mithya.* And you also have that capacity. You take alcohol and what happens? The whole world becomes a *viparyaya;* the whole world becomes false. You start seeing things that are not there.

What has happened? Alcohol cannot create these things, alcohol is doing something within your body and brain. The alcohol starts working the center that Patanjali calls *viparyaya.* The mind has a center that can pervert anything. Once that center starts functioning, everything is perverted.

I am reminded:

Once it happened that Mulla Nasruddin and his friend were drinking in a pub. They came out completely drunk—and Nasruddin was an old, experienced drinker. The other was new, so the other was affected more. So the other asked, "Now I cannot see, I cannot hear, I cannot even walk rightly. How will I reach my home? You tell me, Nasruddin, please direct me. How should I reach my home?"

Nasruddin said, "First you go. After so many steps you will come to a point where there are two ways: One goes to the right, the other goes to the left. You go to the left because that which goes to the right doesn't exist. I have been many times on that right path, but now I am an experienced man. You will see two paths. Choose the left one; don't choose the right. That right path doesn't exist! Many times I have gone on it, and you never reach your home."

Once Nasruddin was teaching his son the first lessons of drinking. The son was curious. He asked, "When is one supposed to stop?"

Nasruddin said, "Look at that table. Four persons are sitting there. When you start seeing eight, stop!"

The boy said, "But father, there are only two persons sitting there!"

Mind has a faculty, and that faculty functions when you are under the influence of a drug or any intoxicant. That faculty Patanjali calls *viparyaya,* wrong knowledge, the center of perversion. Exactly opposite to it is a center that you don't know. Exactly opposite to it is a center, and if you meditate deeply, silently, that other center will start functioning. That center is called *praman,* right knowledge. Through the functioning of that center, whatsoever is known is right.

What you know is not the question; *from where* you know is the question.

That's why all the religions have been against alcohol. It is not on any moralistic grounds, no. It is because alcohol influences the center of perversion. And every religion is for meditation because meditation means creating more and more stillness, becoming more and more silent. Alcohol goes on doing quite the opposite; it makes you more and more agitated, excited, disturbed. A trembling enters within you. The drunkard cannot even walk rightly. His balance is lost. Not only in the body but also in the mind balance is lost.

When you gain the inner balance and there is no trembling, when the whole body-mind has become still, then the center of right knowledge starts functioning. Through that center, whatsoever is known is true.

Meditation means gaining the inner balance. When you gain the inner balance and there is no trembling, when the whole body-mind has become still, then the center of right knowledge starts functioning. Through that center, whatsoever is known is true.

Where are you? You are not alcoholics, and you are not meditators, so you must be somewhere between the two. You are not in any center. You are between these two centers of wrong knowledge and right knowledge. That's why you are confused.

Sometimes you have glimpses. You lean a little toward the right knowledge center, then certain glimpses come to you. You lean toward the other center, which is of perversion, then perversion enters you. And everything is mixed, you are in chaos. That's why either you will have to become meditators, or you will have to become alcoholics because the confusion is too much.

And these are the two ways. If you lose yourself into intoxication, then you are at ease. At least you have gained a center—maybe of wrong knowledge, but you are centered. The whole world may say you are wrong. But you don't think so; you think the whole world is wrong. At least in those moments of unconsciousness you are centered. Centered in the wrong center, but you are happy because even centering in the wrong center gives a certain happiness. You enjoy it; hence alcohol has so much appeal.

Governments have been fighting alcohol and drugs for centuries. Laws have been made, prohibition and everything, but nothing helps. Unless humanity becomes meditative, nothing can help. People will go on; they will find new ways and new means to get intoxicated. They cannot be prevented, and the more you try to prevent them, the greater the appeal.

America did it and had to turn back. They tried their best, but when alcohol was prohibited, even more alcohol was used. They tried and they failed. India was trying after independence, and it failed. It seems useless.

Unless man changes inwardly, you cannot enforce any prohibition. It is impossible because then people will go mad. This is their way to remain sane. For a few hours the person becomes drugged, "stoned," and then he is OK. Then there is no misery; then there is no anguish. The misery will come, the anguish will come, but at least it is postponed. Tomorrow morning the misery will be there, the anguish will be there, and he will have to face it. But by the evening he can hope again—he will take a drink and be at ease.

These are the two alternatives. If you are not meditative, then sooner or later you will have to find some drug. And there are subtle drugs. Alcohol is not very subtle, it is very gross. There are subtle drugs. Sex may become a drug for you, and through sex you may be just losing your consciousness. You can use anything as a drug.

Only meditation can help. Why? Because meditation gives you centering at the center that Patanjali calls *praman*.

Why is there so much emphasis by every Eastern religion on meditation? Meditation must be doing some inner miracle. This is the miracle: Meditation helps you to turn on the light of right knowledge. Then wherever you move, wherever your focus moves, whatsoever is known is true.

Buddha has been asked thousands and thousands of questions. One day somebody asked him, "We come with new questions. We have barely even put the question before you, and you start answering. You never think about it. How does this happen?"

Buddha said, "It is not a question of thinking. You ask the question, and I simply look at it, and whatsoever is true is revealed. It is not a question of thinking and brooding about it. The answer is not coming as a logical syllogism; it is just a focusing of the right center."

Buddha is like a torch. So wherever the torch moves, it reveals—whatever the question, that is not the point. Buddha has the light, and whenever that light comes to any question, the answer will be revealed. The answer will come out of that light. It is a simple phenomenon, a revelation.

When somebody asks you a question, you have to think about it. But how can you think if you don't know? If you know, there is no need to think. If you don't know, what will you do? You will search in your memory, you will find many clues. You will just do a patchwork. You don't know, really; otherwise the response would have been immediate.

I have heard about one teacher:

A woman teacher in a primary school, she asked the children, "Have you got any questions?"

One small boy stood and said, "I have one question, and I have been waiting—whenever you asked, I was going to ask: What is the weight of the whole earth?"

The teacher became disturbed because she had never thought about it, never read about it. What is the weight of the whole earth? So she played a trick that teachers know—they have to play tricks—and said, "Yes, the question is significant. Now, tomorrow, everybody has to find the answer." She needed time. "So tomorrow I will ask the question. Whoever brings the right answer, there will be a present for him."

All the children searched and searched, but they couldn't find the answer. The teacher ran to the library. The whole night she searched, and only just by the morning could she find the weight of the earth. She was very happy. She came back to school, and the children were exhausted. They said they couldn't find the answer: "We asked Mom, and we asked Dad, and we asked everybody. Nobody knows. This question seems to be so difficult!"

The teacher laughed, and she said, "This is not difficult. I know the answer, but I was just trying to see whether you could find it or not. This is the weight of the earth . . ."

The small child who had raised the question stood again, and he said, "With people—or without?"

Now the same situation . . .

You cannot put Buddha in such a situation. It is not a question of finding an answer somewhere; it is not really a question of answering you. Your question is just an excuse. When you put forth a question, he simply moves his light toward that question, and whatsoever is revealed is revealed. He answers *you;* that's a deep response of his right center, *praman.*

Patanjali says there are five modifications of the mind. One is right knowledge. If this center of right knowledge starts functioning in you, you will become a sage, a saint. You will become religious. Before that you cannot become religious.

That's why Jesus and Mohammed look mad—because they don't argue; they don't put their case logically, they simply assert. You ask Jesus, "Are you really the only son of God?" He says, "Yes." And if you ask him to prove it, he will laugh. He will say, "There is no need to prove anything. I know that this is the case; this is self-evident." To us it looks illogical. This man seems to be neurotic, claiming something without any proof.

If this *praman,* this center of *prama,* this center of right knowledge starts functioning, you will be the same! You can assert, but you cannot prove. How can you prove? If you are in love, how can you prove that you are in love? You can simply assert. You have pain in your leg; how can you prove that you have pain? You simply assert, "I have pain." You know it somewhere inside. That knowing is enough.

Ramakrishna was asked, "Is there a God?"

He said yes.

He was asked, "Then prove it."

He said, "There is no need. I *know.* To me there is no need. To you there is a need, so you search. Nobody could prove it for me, and I cannot prove it for you. I had to seek; I had to find. And I have found: God is!"

This is the functioning of the right center.

So Ramakrishna or Jesus look absurd; they are claiming certain things without giving any proof. But, really, they are not claiming; they are not claiming anything. Certain things are revealed to them because they have a new center functioning, which you don't have. And because you don't have it, you want proof.

Remember, wanting proof is evidence that you don't have an inner feeling of anything—everything has to be proved, even love has to be proved. And people go on . . . I know many couples. The husband goes on proving that he loves the wife, and he has not convinced her, and the wife goes on proving that she loves, and she has not convinced the husband. They remain unconvinced, and the conflict remains, and they go on feeling that the other has not proved their love.

Lovers go on searching. They create situations in which the other has to prove that he or she loves. And by and by both get bored—this futile effort to prove, and nothing can be proved. How can you prove love? You can give presents—but nothing is proved. You can kiss and hug, and you can sing, you can dance, but nothing is proved. You may be just pretending.

This first modification of the mind is right knowledge. Meditation leads to this modification. And when you can rightly know, and there is no need to prove, only then can mind be dropped, not before that. When there is no need to prove, the mind is not needed—because mind is a logical instrument. You need it every moment. You have to think, to find out what is wrong and what is right. Every moment there are choices and alternatives. You have to choose. Only when *praman* functions, when right knowledge functions, can you drop the mind because now choosing has no meaning. You move choicelessly, and whatsoever is right is revealed to you.

The definition of the sage is one who never chooses. He never chooses good against bad. He simply moves toward the direction of the good. It is just like sunflowers. When the sun is in the east, the flower moves to the east. It never chooses. When the sun moves to the west, the flower moves to the west. It simply moves with the sun. It has not chosen to move; it has not decided, it has not taken a decision that "Now I should move because the sun has moved to the west."

> The definition of the sage is one who never chooses. He never chooses good against bad. He simply moves toward the direction of the good.

A sage is just like a sunflower. Wherever is good he simply moves. So whatever he does is good. The Upanishads say, "Don't judge the sages. Your ordinary measurements won't do." You have to do good against the bad; the sage has nothing to choose. He simply moves. And you cannot change him because it is not a question of alternatives. If you say, "This is bad," he will say, "OK, it may be bad, but this is how I move. This is how my being flows."

Those who know—and people in the days of the Upanishads knew—have decided, "We will not judge a sage. Once a person has come to be centered in himself, when a person has achieved meditation, once a person has become silent and the mind has been dropped, he is beyond our morality, beyond tradition. He is beyond our limitations. If we can follow, we can follow him. If we cannot follow, we are helpless. But nothing can be done, and we should not judge."

If right knowledge functions, if your mind has taken the modification of right knowledge, you will become religious.

Look, it is totally different. Patanjali doesn't say if you go to the mosque, to the temple, if you do some ritual, you pray. . . . No, that's not religion. You have to make your right-knowledge center function. So whether you go to the temple or not is immaterial; it doesn't matter. If your right-knowledge center functions, whatever you do is prayer, and wherever you go is a temple.

Kabir has said, "Wherever I go, I find you, my God. Wherever I move, I move into you, I stumble upon you. And whatever I do, even walking, eating, it is prayer." Kabir says, "This spontaneity is my *samadhi.* Just to be spontaneous is my meditation."

The second modification of the mind is wrong knowledge. If your center of wrong knowledge is functioning, then whatever you do you will do wrongly, and whatever you choose you will choose wrongly. Whatever you decide will be wrong because *you* are not deciding, the wrong center is.

There are people who feel very unfortunate because whatever they do goes wrong. And they try not to do wrong again, but that's not going to help because the *center* has to be changed. Their minds function in a wrong way. They may think that they are doing good, but they will do bad. With all their good wishes or intentions, they cannot help; they are helpless.

> Mulla Nasruddin used to visit a saint. He visited for many, many days. And the saint was a silent one; he would not speak. Then Mulla Nasruddin had to say something; he had to ask, "I have been coming again and again, waiting for you to say something, and you have not said anything. And unless you speak, I cannot understand. So just

give me a message for my life, a direction so that I can move in that direction."

So that Sufi sage said, "*Neki kar kuyen may dal:* Do good, and throw it in the well." It is one of the oldest Sufi sayings: "Do good and throw it in the well." It means do good, and forget it immediately; don't carry the thought that "I have done good."

So next day Mulla Nasruddin helped one old woman to cross the road . . . and then he pushed her into the well! *Neki kar kuyen may dal:* Do good and throw it in the well.

If your wrong center is functioning, whatsoever you do . . . You can read the Koran, you can read the Gita, and you will find meanings in them—Krishna will be shocked, Mohammed will be shocked, to see that you can find such meanings.

Mahatma Gandhi wrote his autobiography with the intention that it would help people. Then many letters came to him because he describes his sex life. He was honest, one of the most honest men, so he wrote everything—whatever had happened in his past, how he was too indulgent the day his father was dying and he couldn't sit by his side. Even that day he had to go with his wife to bed.

And doctors had said, "This is the last night. Your father cannot survive the morning. He will be dead by the morning." But just about twelve or one in the night, Gandhi started feeling sexual desire. The father was sleepy, so Gandhi slipped away and went to his wife, indulged in sex. And the wife was pregnant; it was the ninth month. The father was dying—the father died in the night—and the child died the moment he was born. So for his whole life, Gandhi had a deep repentance that he hadn't been with his dying father because sex was such an obsession.

So he wrote everything; he was honest—and just to help others. But many letters started coming to him, and those letters shocked him. Many people wrote, "Your autobiography is such that we have become more sexual than before just by reading it. Just reading through your autobiography we have become more sexual and indulgent. It is erotic."

If the wrong center is functioning, then nothing can be done. Whatever you do or read, however you behave, it will be wrong. You will move to the wrong; you have a center that is forcing you to move toward the wrong. You can go to Buddha, but you will see something wrong in him. Immediately! You cannot meet Buddha; you will see something wrong immediately. You have a focus for the wrong, a deep urge to find wrong anywhere and everywhere.

This modification of the mind Patanjali calls *viparyaya,* which means "perversion." You pervert everything. You interpret everything in such a way that it becomes a perversion.

Omar Khayyam writes, "I have heard that God is compassionate." This is beautiful. Mohammedans go on repeating, "God is *rehmaṇ,* compassion; *rahim,* compassion." They go on repeating it continually. So Omar Khayyam says, "If he really is compassionate, if he is compassion, then there is no need to be afraid. I can go on committing sin. If God is compassion, then what is the fear? I can commit whatsoever I want, and he is compassion—so whenever I will stand before him, I will say, *Rahim, rehman*: Oh, God of compassion, I have sinned, but you are compassion. If you are really compassion, then have compassion on me." So he goes on drinking, he goes on committing whatever he thinks is sin. He has interpreted in a very perverted way.

All over the world people have done that. In India we say, "If you go to the Ganges, if you bathe in the Ganges, your sins will dissolve." It is a beautiful concept in itself. It shows many things. It shows that sin is not something very deep; it is just like dust on you. So don't get too obsessed by it, don't feel guilty. It is just dust, and you remain pure inside. Even bathing in the Ganges can help.

This is just to show you not to become so obsessed with sin as Christianity has become. Guilt has become so burdensome. So even just taking a bath in the Ganges will help. Don't be so afraid. But how have we interpreted it? We say, "Then it is OK. Go on committing sin. And after a while, when you feel now you have committed many, give the Ganges a chance to purify you; then come back and commit sins again." This is the center of perversion.

The third modification of the mind is imagination. Mind has the faculty to imagine. It is good, it is beautiful. All that is beautiful has come through imagination. Art, dance, music—everything that is beautiful has come through imagination. But everything that is ugly has also come through imagination. Hitler, Mao, Mussolini—they have all come through imagination.

Hitler imagined a world of supermen, and he believed in Friedrich Nietzsche, who said, "Destroy all those who are weak. Destroy all those who are not superior. Leave only supermen on the earth." So Hitler destroyed people. Just imagination, just utopian imagination—to think that just by destroying the weak, just by destroying the ugly, just by destroying the physically crippled, you will have a beautiful world. But the very destruction is the ugliest thing in the world possible—the very destruction.

But he was working through imagination. He had an imagination, a utopian imagination—the most imaginative man! Hitler was one of the most imaginative people, and his imagination became so fantastic and so mad that for his imaginative world, he tried to destroy this world completely. His imagination had gone mad.

Imagination can give you poetry and music and art, and imagination can also give you madness. It depends on how you use it. All the great scientific discoveries have been through imagination—people who could imagine, who could imagine the impossible. Now we can fly into the air, now we can go to the moon. These are deep imaginations. Man has been imagining for centuries, millennia, how to fly, how to go to the moon. Every child is born with the desire to go to the moon, to catch the moon. But we reached it! Through imagination comes creativity, but through imagination also comes destruction.

> Imagination can give you poetry and music and art, and imagination can also give you madness. It depends on how you use it.

Patanjali says imagination is the third mode of the mind. You can use it in a wrong way, and then it will destroy you. You can use it in a right way, and then there are imaginative meditations. They start with imagination, but by and by imagination becomes subtler and subtler and subtler. And ultimately imagination is dropped, and you are face to face with the truth.

All Christian and Mohammedan meditations are basically through imagination. First you have to imagine something. And then you go on imagining it, and then through imagination you create an atmosphere around you. You try it, you see through imagination what is possible. Even the impossible is possible.

If you think you are beautiful, if you imagine you are beautiful, a certain beauty will start happening to your body. So whenever a man says to a woman, "You are beautiful," the woman has changed immediately. She may not have been beautiful before this moment—just homely, ordinary. But this man has given imagination to her. So every woman who is loved becomes more beautiful; every man who is loved becomes more beautiful. A person who is not loved may be beautiful but becomes ugly because he cannot imagine, she cannot imagine. And if imagination is not there, you shrink.

Emile Coué, one of the great psychologists of the West, helped millions of people to be cured of many, many diseases just through imagination. His formula was very simple. He would say, "Just start feeling that you are OK. Just go on repeating inside the mind, 'I am getting better and better. Every day I am getting better.' At night while you fall asleep, go on thinking you are healthy, and you are getting healthier every moment, and by the morning you will be the healthiest person in the world. Go on imagining." And he helped millions of people. Even incurable diseases were cured. It looked like a miracle; it is not. It is just a basic law: Your mind follows imagination.

Now psychologists say that if you say to children that they are slow, that they are dull, they become dull. You force them to be dull. You give their imagination the suggestion that they are dull. Many experiments have been done. Say to a child, "You are dull. You cannot do anything; you cannot solve this mathematical problem." And give him the problem and tell him, "Now try," he will not be able to solve it. You have closed the door. Say to the child, "You are intelligent, and I have not seen any boy as intelligent as you are. For your age you are exceptionally intelligent. You show many potentialities; you can solve any problem. Now try this. . . ." And he will be able to solve it. You have given imagination to him.

Now these are scientific proofs, scientific discoveries that whatsoever imagination catches, it becomes a seed. Whole generations have been changed, whole ages, whole countries have been changed just through imagination.

Go to Punjab. . . . I was traveling once from Delhi to Manali. My driver was a Sikh, a *sardar.* The road was dangerous, and the car was very big, and many times the driver became afraid. Many times he would say, "I cannot go ahead. We will have to go back." We tried in every way to persuade him. At one point he became so afraid that he stopped the car, got out, and said, "No! Now I cannot move from here. It is dangerous." He said, "It may not be dangerous for you; you may be ready to die. But I am not—I want to go back."

By chance one of my friends, who is also a *sardar* and was a big police official, was also coming on that road. He had been following me to attend a meditation camp in Manali. His car came alongside, so I told him, "Do something! The man has run out of the car."

The police official went to the driver and he said, "You being a *sardar* and a Sikh—and a coward? Get into the car." The man immediately came into the car and started driving.

So I asked him, "What happened?"

He said, "Now he has touched my ego. He said, 'You are a *sardar*? (*Sardar* means "leader of men.") A Sikh and a coward?' He has touched my imagination, he has touched my pride. Now we can go. Dead or alive—but we will reach Manali."

And this has not happened just with one man. If you go to Punjab, you will see that it has happened with millions. Look at the Hindus of Punjab and the Sikhs of Punjab. Their blood is the same; they belong to the same race. Five hundred years ago all were Hindus. And then a different type of race, a military race, was born. Just by growing a beard, just by changing your face you cannot become brave. But you can! Imagination . . .

Nanak gave the imagination to the Sikhs: "You are a different type of race. You are unconquerable." And once they believed it, once that imagination started to work in the Punjab, within five hundred years a new race, totally different from Punjabi Hindus, came into being. Nothing is different in reality. But in India, no one is braver than they. Two world wars have proved that on the whole of the earth, Sikhs have no comparison. They can fight fearlessly.

Imagination works. It can make a brave man out of you, or it can make a coward.

What happened? Their imagination created a milieu around them. They feel that just by being Sikhs, they are different. Imagination works. It can make a brave man out of you, or it can make a coward.

I have heard:

Mulla Nasruddin was sitting in a pub drinking. He was not a brave man—he was one of the most cowardly. But alcohol gave him courage. Then a man, a giant of a man, entered the pub—ferocious looking, dangerous, he looked like a murderer. At any other time, if he had been in his senses, Mulla Nasruddin would have been afraid. But now he was drunk, so he was not afraid at all.

That ferocious-looking man came near Mulla, and seeing that he was not afraid at all he stomped on his foot. Mulla got angry, furious, and he said, "What are you doing? Are you doing that on purpose, or it is just a sort of joke?"

But by this time, feeling the pain in his foot, Mulla was

brought back from his alcohol-induced bravery. He came to his senses. And he had already said, "What are you doing—was it on purpose or was it just a sort of joke?"

The man said, "On purpose."

Mulla Nasruddin said, "Then thank you because I don't like such types of jokes. On purpose it is OK."

Patanjali says imagination is the mind's third faculty. You go on imagining, and if you wrongly imagine, you can create delusions around you, illusions, dreams—you can be lost in them. LSD and other drugs, they work on this center. So whatever inside potential you have, your LSD trip will help you to develop it. Nothing is certain. If you have happy imaginations, the drug trip will be a happy trip, a high. If you have miserable imaginations, nightmarish imaginations, the trip is going to be bad.

That's why many people report contradictorily. Huxley says that LSD can become a key to the door of heaven, and Rheiner says it is the ultimate hell. It depends on you. LSD cannot do anything; it simply jumps on your center of imagination and starts functioning chemically there. If you have an imagination of the nightmarish type, then you will develop that, and you will pass through hell. And if you are addicted to beautiful dreams, you may reach heaven. This imagination can function either as a hell or as heaven. You can use it to go completely insane.

What has happened to madmen in the madhouses? They have used their imagination, and they have used it in such a way that they are engulfed by it. A madman may be sitting alone, but he is talking aloud to someone. He not only talks, he also answers. He questions, he answers, he also speaks for the other, who is absent. You may think that he is mad, but he is talking to a real person. In his imagination the person is real, and he cannot judge what is imaginary and what is real.

Children cannot judge, so many times children may lose their toy in a dream, and then they will weep in the morning, "Where is my toy?" They cannot judge that a dream is a dream, and reality is reality. But they have not lost anything, they were just dreaming. Boundaries are blurred; they don't know where dreaming ends and where reality starts. A madman is also blurred. He doesn't know what is real, what is unreal.

If imagination is used rightly, then you will know that this is imagination, and you will remain alert. You can enjoy it, but you will know it is not real.

When people meditate, many things happen through their imagination. They start seeing lights, colors, visions, talking to God himself or moving with Jesus or dancing with Krishna. These are imaginative things, and a meditator has to remember that these are functions of the imagination. You can enjoy it; nothing is wrong in these things—they are fun. Don't think that they are real.

If imagination is used rightly, then you will know that this is imagination, and you will remain alert. You can enjoy it, but you will know it is not real.

Remember that only the witnessing consciousness is real, nothing else. Whatsoever happens may be beautiful, worth enjoying—enjoy it. It is beautiful to dance with Krishna; nothing is wrong in it. Dance! Enjoy it! But remember continuously that this is imagination, a beautiful dream. Don't be lost in it. If you get lost, then imagination has become dangerous. Many religious people are just living in imagination. And they move in imagination and waste their lives.

The fourth modification of the mind is sleep. Sleep means unconsciousness as far as your outward-moving consciousness is concerned. The consciousness has gone deep into itself. Activity has stopped; conscious activity has stopped. The mind is not functioning—sleep is a nonfunctioning of the mind. If you are dreaming, then it is not sleep; you are just in the middle, in the waking and the sleep. You have left the waking and you have not entered sleep; you are just in the middle.

Sleep means a state totally without content—no activity, no movement in the mind. The mind has completely been absorbed, relaxed. This sleep is beautiful; it is life-giving. You can use it, and if you know how to use this sleep, it can become *samadhi* because *samadhi* and sleep are not very different. The only difference is that in *samadhi* you will be aware. Everything else will be the same. In sleep everything is the same, only you are not aware. You are in the same bliss into which Buddha entered, in which Ramakrishna lives, in which Jesus has made his home. In deep sleep you are in the same blissful state, but you are not aware. So in the morning you feel the night has been good. In the morning you feel refreshed, vital, rejuvenated. In the morning you feel that the night was just beautiful—but this is only an afterglow. You don't know what has happened, what really happened. You were not aware.

Sleep can be used in two ways. One is just as a natural rest—but you have even lost that. People are not really going into sleep. They continuously dream. Sometimes for very few seconds they touch sleep. They touch it, and they again start dreaming. The silence of sleep, the blissful music of sleep, has become unknown. You have destroyed it. Even natural sleep is destroyed. You are so agitated and excited that the mind cannot fall completely into oblivion.

But Patanjali says natural sleep is good for the health of the body, and if you can become alert in sleep, it can become *samadhi,* it can become a spiritual phenomenon. So there are techniques for how sleep can become an awakening. The *Bhagavad Gita* says that the yogi doesn't sleep even while he is asleep. He remains alert; something inside goes on being aware. The whole body falls into sleep, the mind falls into sleep, but the witnessing remains. Someone is watching—a watcher in the tower continues—then sleep becomes *samadhi.* It becomes the ultimate ecstasy.

Natural sleep is good for the health of the body, and if you can become alert in sleep, it can become a spiritual phenomenon.

Memory is the fifth—and last—modification of the mind. That, too, can be used or misused. If memory is misused, it creates confusion. Really, you may remember something, but you cannot be certain whether it happened that way or not. Your memory is not reliable. You may add many things to it; imagination may enter into it. You may delete many things from it, you may do many things to it. When you say, "This is my memory," it is a refined and changed thing; it is not real.

Everybody says, "My childhood was just paradise," and yet look at children! These children will also say later on that their childhood was paradise, and right now they are suffering. Every child hankers to grow up quickly, to become an adult. Every child thinks that adults are enjoying all that is worth enjoying. They are powerful, they can do everything, and the child is helpless. Children think that they are suffering. But these children will grow as you have grown, and then later on they will say that childhood was beautiful, just a paradise.

Your memory is not reliable; you are imagining. You are just creating your past, you are not true to it. You drop many things from it—all that was ugly, all that was sad, all that was painful you drop; all that was beautiful you keep. All that was a support to your ego you remember, and you drop all that was not a support, you forget it. So everybody has a great storehouse of dropped memories. And whatsoever you say is not true, you cannot truly remember. All your centers are confused, and they enter into each other and disturb things.

Right memory—Buddha has used the words "right memory" for meditation. Patanjali says if memory is right, that means one has to be totally honest to oneself. Then and only then can memory be right. Whatsoever has happened, bad or good, don't change it. Know it as it is.

> Knowing one's past as it is will change your whole life. If you rightly know your past as it is, you will not want to repeat it in the future.

It is very hard; it is arduous! You choose and change. Knowing one's past as it is will change your whole life. If you rightly know your past as it is, you will not want to repeat it in the future. Right now everybody is thinking of how to repeat the past in a modified form—but if you know your past exactly as it was, you will not want to repeat it. Right memory will give you the impetus to be free from *all* lives. And if memory is right, then you can go even into your past lives. If you are honest, then you can go into past lives—

and then you will have only one desire: to find out how to transcend all this nonsense.

You think the past was beautiful, and you think the future is going to be beautiful; only the present is wrong. But the past was present just a few days before, and the future will become present a few days hence. Each time, every present is wrong—and all past is beautiful and all future is beautiful? This is wrong memory. Look directly. Don't change anything. Look at the past as it was.

But we are dishonest.

Every man hates his father, but if you ask anybody, he will say, "I love my father. I honor my father above anything." Every woman hates her mother—but ask, and every woman will say, "My mother is just wonderful." This is wrong memory.

Khalil Gibran has a story. He says that one night a mother and daughter were awakened suddenly because of a noise. They both were sleepwalkers, and at the time the sudden noise happened in the neighborhood, they were both walking in the garden, asleep. They were somnambulists.

In her sleep the mother was saying to the daughter, "Because of you, you bitch, because of you, my youth is lost. You destroyed me. And now anybody who comes to the house looks at you. Nobody looks at me." This deep jealousy comes to every mother when the daughter is young and beautiful—it happens to every mother, but it is hidden inside.

And the daughter was saying, "You old rotten . . . Because of you I cannot enjoy life. You are the hindrance. Everywhere you are the hindrance, the obstacle. I cannot love, I cannot enjoy . . ."

And suddenly because of the noise they were both awakened.

And the old woman said, "My child, what are you doing here? You may catch cold. Come inside."

And the daughter said, "But what are you doing here? You were not feeling well, and this is a cold night. Come, Mother. Come to bed."

The first dialogue was coming from the unconscious. Now they have awakened, and they are again pretending. Now the unconscious has receded; the conscious has come in. Now they are hypocrites.

Your conscious is hypocrisy. To be truly honest with one's own memories, one will have to really pass through arduous effort. You have to be true, whatsoever the cost. You have to be nakedly true—you have to know what you really think about your father, about your mother, about your brother, about your sister. Really. And whatever you have in your past, don't mix it, don't change it, don't polish it; let it be as it is. If this happens, then, Patanjali says, this will be freedom. You will drop it. The whole thing is nonsense, and you will not want to project it again into the future.

And then you will not be a hypocrite. You will be real, true, sincere—you will become authentic. And when you become authentic, you become like a rock. Nothing can change you; nothing can create confusion. You become like a sword. You can always cut away whatsoever is wrong; you can divide the right from the wrong. Then a clarity of mind is achieved. That clarity can lead you toward meditation; that clarity can become the basic ground to grow—to grow beyond.

3

CONSTANT EFFORT IS THE KEY

The first state of vairagya, *desirelessness—cessation from self-indulgence in the thirst for sensuous pleasures, with conscious effort.*
The last state of vairagya, *desirelessness—cessation of all desiring by knowing the innermost nature of* purusha, *the supreme self.*

ABHYASA and *vairagya*—constant inner practice and desirelessness—these are the two foundation stones of Patanjali's yoga. Constant inner effort is needed not because something has to be achieved but because of wrong habits. The fight is not against nature, the fight is against habits. The nature is there, available to flow within you every moment, to become one with it, but you have a wrong pattern of habits. Those habits create barriers. The fight is against these habits—and unless they are destroyed, your inherent nature cannot flow, cannot move, cannot reach its destiny.

So remember the first thing: The struggle is not against nature; the struggle is against wrong nurture, wrong habits. You are not fighting yourself, you are fighting something else that has become affixed to you. If this is not understood rightly, then your whole effort can go in a wrong direction. You may start fighting with yourself, and once you start fighting with yourself, you are fighting a losing battle. You can never be victorious. Who will be victorious, and who will be defeated? Because you

> The struggle is not against nature; the struggle is against wrong nurture, wrong habits. You are not fighting yourself, you are fighting something else that has become affixed to you. If this is not understood rightly, then your whole effort can go in a wrong direction.

are both: The one who is fighting and the one with whom you are fighting are the same.

If both my hands start fighting, who is going to win? Once you start fighting with yourself you are lost. And so many people, in their endeavors, in their seeking for spiritual truth, fall into that error. They become victims of this error; they start fighting with themselves. If you fight with yourself, you will go more and more insane. You will be more and more divided: split. You will become schizophrenic.

This is what is happening in the West. Christianity has taught—not Christ, but Christianity—to fight with oneself, to condemn oneself, to deny oneself. Christianity has created a great division between the lower and the higher. There is nothing lower and nothing higher in you, but Christianity talks about the lower self and the higher self, or the body and the soul, but somehow Christianity divides you and creates a fight. This fight is going to be endless; it will not lead you anywhere. The ultimate result can only be self-destruction, a schizophrenic chaos. That's what is happening in the West.

Yoga never divides you. But still there is a fight. The fight is not against your nature; on the contrary, the fight is *for* your nature. You have accumulated many habits. Those habits are the achievement of many lives' wrong patterns. And because of those wrong patterns your nature cannot move spontaneously, cannot flow spontaneously, and cannot reach its destiny. These habits have to be destroyed—and these are only habits! They may look like nature to you because you are so addicted to them. You may have become identified with them, but they are not you.

This distinction has to be clearly maintained in the mind, otherwise you can misinterpret Patanjali. Whatever has come into you from without and is wrong has to be destroyed so that what is within you can flow, can flower. *Abhyasa,* constant inner practice, is against habits.

The second thing, the second foundation stone, is *vairagya,* desirelessness. That too can lead you in the wrong direction. And remember, these are not rules, these are simple directions. When I say these are not rules, I mean they are not to be followed like an obsession. They have to be understood—the meaning, the significance—and the significance has to be carried into your life. It is going to be different for everyone, so it is not a fixed rule. You are not to follow it dogmatically. You have to understand its significance and allow it to grow within you. The flowering is going to be different with each individual. So these are not dead, dogmatic rules, these are simple directions. They indicate the direction; they don't give you the detail.

I remember once that Mulla Nasruddin was working as a doorkeeper in a museum. The day he was appointed, he asked, "What rules have to be followed?" So he was given the book of the rules to be followed by the doorkeeper. He memorized them; he took every care not to forget a single detail. And the first day he was on duty, the first visitor came. Nasruddin told the visitor to leave his umbrella outside with him at the door. The visitor was amazed. He said, "But I don't have any umbrella."

So Nasruddin said, "In that case, you will have to go back. Bring an umbrella, because this is the rule. Unless a visitor leaves his umbrella outside with me, he cannot be allowed in."

There are many people who are rule obsessed. They follow blindly. Patanjali is not interested in giving you rules. Whatsoever he says are simple directions—not to be followed, but to be understood. The following will come out of that understanding. And the reverse cannot happen. If you follow the rules, understanding will not come. If you understand the rules, the following will come automatically as a shadow.

There are many people who are rule obsessed. They follow blindly. Patanjali is not interested in giving you rules. Whatsoever he says are simple directions—not to be followed, but to be understood.

Desirelessness is a direction. If you follow it as a rule, then you will start killing your desires. Many have done that—millions have done that. They start killing their desires. Of course, this is mathematical, this is logical. If desirelessness is to be achieved, then this is the best way: to kill all desires. Then you will be without desires.

But you will also be dead. You have followed the rule exactly, but if you kill all desires, you are killing yourself, you are committing suicide. Because desires are not only desires, they are the flow of life energy.

Desirelessness is to be achieved without killing anything. Desirelessness is to be achieved with more life, with more energy—not less. For example, you can kill sex easily if you starve the body because sex and food are deeply related. Food is needed for your survival, for the survival of the individual, and sex is needed for the survival of the race, of the species. They are both food in a way. Without food the individual cannot survive, and without sex the race cannot survive. But the individual is primary. If the individual cannot survive, then there is no question of the race surviving.

So if you starve your body, if you give so little food to your body that the energy created by it is exhausted in day-to-day routine work—your walking, sitting, sleeping—and no extra energy accumulates, then sex will disappear. Because sex can be there only when the individual is gathering extra energy, more than he needs for his survival; then the body can think of the survival of the race. If you are in danger, then the body simply forgets about sex. Hence so much attraction for fasting because if you fast, sex disappears. But this is not desirelessness. This is just becoming more and more dead, less and less alive.

Monks in India have been fasting continually just for this end because if you fast continually and you are constantly on a starvation diet, sex disappears. Nothing else is needed—no transformation of the mind, no transformation of the inner energy. Simply starving helps. Then you become habituated to the starvation. And if you do it for years, you will simply forget that sex exists. No energy is created; no energy moves to the sex center. There is no energy to move! The person exists just as a dead being. There is no sex.

But this is not what Patanjali means. This is not a desireless state, it is simply an impotent state; energy is not there. Give proper food to the body—and you may have starved the body for thirty or forty years—and sex reappears immediately. You are not changed; the sex has just been hiding there, waiting for energy to flow. Whenever energy flows it will become alive again.

So what is the criterion to judge? The criterion has to be remembered. Be more alive, be more filled with energy, be vital, and become desireless. Only then, if your desirelessness makes you more alive, have you followed the right direction. If it makes you simply a dead person, you have only followed the rule. It is easy to follow the rule because no intelligence is required. It is easy to follow the rule because simple tricks can do it. Fasting is a simple trick. Nothing much is implied in it; no wisdom is going to come out of it.

There was one experiment in Oxford. For thirty days a group of twenty students was totally starved—young, healthy boys. After the seventh or eighth day they started losing interest in girls. Nude pictures were shown to them, and they were indifferent. And this indifference was not just bodily, even their minds were not interested—because now there are methods to judge the mind. Whenever a young, healthy boy looks at a nude picture of a girl, the pupils of his eyes become bigger. They open more to receive the nude figure. And you cannot control your pupils; this is not voluntary. So you may *say* that you are not interested in sex, but a nude picture will reveal whether you are interested or not. And you cannot do anything voluntarily; you cannot control the pupils of your eyes. They expand because something so interesting has come before them that they open more; the shutters open more to take more in.

Every effort was made to determine whether these students at Oxford were interested; there was no interest. By and by, the interest declined. Even in their dreams they stopped seeing girls, stopped having sexual dreams. By the second week, the fourteenth or fifteenth day, they were simply dead corpses. Even if a beautiful girl came near, they would not look. If someone told a dirty joke, they would not laugh. For thirty days they were starved, and by the thirtieth day, the whole group was sexless. There was no sex in their minds, in their bodies.

Then food was given to them again. The very first day they became again the same. The next day they were interested, and by the third day, all that starving for thirty days had disappeared. Now not only they were interested, they were *obsessively* interested—as if this gap had helped. For a few weeks they were obsessively sexual, only thinking of girls and nothing else. Food was in the body, so girls became important again. But this has been done in many countries all over the world. Many religions have followed this fasting, and then people start thinking they have gone beyond sex.

You can go beyond sex, but fasting is not the way. That's a trick. And this can be done in every way. If you are on fast, you will be less angry, and if you become habituated to fasting, then many things will simply drop from your life because the base has dropped. Food is the base. When you have more energy, you move in more dimensions. When you are filled with overflowing energy, your overflowing energy leads you into many, many desires. Desires are nothing but outlets for energy.

So two ways are possible. One is that your desire goes; the energy remains. The other, energy is removed; desire remains.

Energy can be removed very easily. You can simply be operated upon, castrated, and then sex disappears. Some hormones can be removed from your body. And that's what fasting is doing—some hormones disappear, and then you can become sexless. But this is not the goal of Patanjali. Patanjali says that energy should remain and the desire disappear. Only when desire disappears and you are filled with energy can you achieve that blissful state that yoga aims to reach. A dead person cannot reach to the beyond. The beyond can be attained only through overflowing energy, abundant energy, an ocean of energy.

So this is the second thing to remember always: Don't destroy energy, destroy desire. It will be difficult. It is going to be hard, arduous, because it needs a total transformation of your being. But Patanjali is for it. So he divides his *vairagya,* his desirelessness, in two steps.

We will enter the sutra.

The first:

> ***The first state of* vairagya, *desirelessness—cessation from self-indulgence in the thirst for sensuous pleasures, with conscious effort.***

Many things are implied and have to be understood. For one, the indulgence in sensuous pleasures—why do you ask for sensuous pleasures? Why does the mind constantly think about indulgence? Why do you move again and again in the same patterns of indulgence?

For Patanjali, and for all those who have known, the reason is that you are not blissful inwardly; hence the desire for pleasure. The pleasure-oriented mind means that as you are, in yourself, you are unhappy. That's why you go on seeking happiness somewhere else.

A person who is unhappy is bound to move into desires. Desires are the way of the unhappy mind to seek happiness. Of course, nowhere can this mind find happiness. At the most he can find few glimpses. Those glimpses appear as pleasure. Pleasure means glimpses of happiness. And the fallacy is that this pleasure-seeking mind thinks these glimpses and pleasures are coming from somewhere else.

It always comes from within.

> Pleasure means glimpses of happiness. And the fallacy is that this pleasure-seeking mind thinks these glimpses and pleasures are coming from somewhere else. It always comes from within.

Let us try to understand. You are in love with a person. You move into sex. Sex gives you a glimpse of pleasure; it gives you a glimpse of happiness. For a single moment you feel at ease. All the miseries have disappeared, all the mental agony is no more. For a single moment you are here and now, you have forgotten all. For a single moment there is no past and no future. Because of this—there is no past and no future, and for a single moment you are here and now—the energy flows from within you. Your inner self flows in this moment, and you have a glimpse of happiness.

But you think that the glimpse is coming from the partner, from the woman or from the man. It is not coming from the woman or from the man. It is coming from you! The other has simply helped you to fall into the present, to fall out of the future and the past. The other has simply helped to bring you to the nowness of this moment.

If you can come to this nowness without sex, by and by sex, will become useless; it will disappear. It will not be a desire then. If you want to move into it, you can move into it as fun but not as a desire. Then there is no obsession in it because you are not dependent on it.

Sit under a tree some day—just in the morning when the sun has not risen because with the sun rising your body is disturbed, and it is difficult to be at peace within. That is why the East has always been meditating before the sunrise. They have called it *brahmamuhurt,* the moments of the divine. And they are right because with the sun, energies rise and start flowing in the old patterns that you have created.

When the sun has not yet come up on the horizon, everything is silent, and nature is fast asleep—the trees are asleep, the birds are asleep, the whole world is asleep. Your body inside is also asleep—you have come to sit under a tree. Everything is silent. Just try to be here in this moment. Don't do anything; don't even meditate. Don't make any effort. Just close your eyes, remain silent in this silence of nature. Suddenly you will have the same glimpse that has been coming to you through sex—or even greater, deeper. Suddenly you will feel a rush of energy flowing from within. And now you cannot be deceived because there is no "other"; it is certainly coming from you. It is certainly flowing from within. Nobody else is giving it to you; you are giving it to yourself.

But the situation is needed—a silence, energy, not in excitement. You are not doing anything, just being there under a tree. And you will have the glimpse. And this will not really be the ordinary pleasure, it will be the happiness—because now you are looking at the right source, the right direction. Once you know it, then through sex you will immediately recognize that the other was just a mirror; you were just reflected in him or in her. And you were the mirror for the other. You were helping each other to fall into the present, to move away from the thinking mind to a nonthinking state of being.

The more the mind is filled with chattering, the more sex has an appeal. In the East, sex was never such an obsession as it has become in the West. Films, stories, novels, poetry, magazines—

everything has become sexual. You cannot sell anything unless you can create sex appeal. If you have to sell a car, you can sell it only as a sex object; if you want to sell toothpaste, you can sell it only through some sex appeal. Nothing can be sold without sex. It seems that only sex has the market; nothing else has any significance. Every significance comes through sex. The whole mind is obsessed with sex.

Why? Why has this never happened before? This is something new in human history. And the reason is that now in the West people are totally absorbed in thoughts—there is no possibility of being here and now except through sex. Sex has remained the only possibility, and even that is going. For the modern man, even this has become possible: that while making love he can think of other things. And once you become capable of making love while at the same time you go on thinking of something else—of your accounts in the bank or you go on talking with a friend or you go on being somewhere else while making love here—sex will also be finished. Then it will just be boring, frustrating, because sex was not the thing. The thing was only because when sexual energy is moving so fast, your mind comes to a stop, and the sex takes over. The energy flows so fast, so vitally, that your ordinary patterns of thinking stop.

I have heard:

> Once it happened that Mulla Nasruddin was passing through a forest. He came upon a skull. Just curious, as he always is, he asked the skull, "What brought you here, sir?"
>
> And he was amazed because the skull said, "Talking brought me here, sir."
>
> Nasruddin couldn't believe it—but he had heard it, so he ran to the court of the king. He told him, "I have seen

a miracle! A skull, a talking skull, lying just near our village in the forest."

The king also couldn't believe it, but he was curious. The whole court followed him, and they went into the forest. Nasruddin went near the skull and again asked the same question: "What brought you here, sir?" But the skull remained silent. He asked again and again and again, but the skull was dead silent.

The king said, "I knew it before, Nasruddin, that you were a liar. But now this is too much. You have played such a joke that you will have to suffer for it." He ordered his guard to cut off Nasruddin's head and throw it near the skull for the ants to eat.

When everybody had gone away—the king, his court—the skull started talking again. And it asked, "What brought you here, sir?"

Nasruddin answered, "Talking brought me here, sir."

Talking has brought man here—that is the situation today. A constantly chattering mind does not allow any happiness, any possibility of happiness because only a silent mind can look within. Only a silent mind can hear the silence, the happiness that is always bubbling there. It is so subtle that with the noise of the mind you cannot hear it.

Only a silent mind can look within. Only a silent mind can hear the silence, the happiness that is always bubbling there. It is so subtle that with the noise of the mind you cannot hear it.

Only in sex does the noise sometimes stop. I say "sometimes"—if you have also become habitual in sex, as husbands and wives become, then the noise never stops. The whole act becomes automatic, and the mind goes on its own. Then sex, too, is a boredom.

Anything has an appeal if it can give you a glimpse. The glimpse may appear to be coming from the outside, but it always comes from within. The outside can only be a mirror. When happiness flowing from within is reflected from the outside, it is called pleasure. This is Patanjali's definition of pleasure: happiness flowing from within, reflected from somewhere outside, with the outside functioning as a mirror. If you think that this happiness is really coming from the outside, it is called pleasure. We are in search of *happiness,* not in search of pleasure. So unless you can have glimpses of happiness, you cannot stop your pleasure-seeking efforts. Indulgence means the search for pleasure.

A conscious effort is needed for two things. One: Whenever you feel a moment of pleasure is there, transform it into a meditative situation. Whenever you feel that you are experiencing pleasure, happy, joyful, close your eyes and look within and see from where it is coming. Don't lose this moment; this is precious. If you are not conscious you may continue to think that it comes from without, and that's the fallacy of the world.

If you are conscious, meditative, if you search for the real source, sooner or later you will come to know that it is flowing from within. Once you know that it always flows from within, that it is something that you already have, indulgence will drop. And this will be the first step of desirelessness. Then you are not seeking, not hankering. You are not killing desires, you are not fighting with desires—you have simply found something greater. Desires don't look so important now. They wither away.

Remember this: Desires are not to be killed and destroyed;

they wither away. You simply neglect them because you have a greater source, and you are magnetically attracted toward it. Now your whole energy is moving inward. The desires are simply neglected. You are not fighting them. If you fight with them, you will never win.

It is just as if you had some stones, colored stones, in your hand, and now suddenly you have come to know about diamonds, and they are lying all about. You throw away the colored stones to create space for the diamonds in your hand. You are not fighting the stones. When diamonds are there, you simply drop the stones. They have lost their meaning.

Desires must lose their meaning. If you fight, the meaning is not lost. In fact, on the contrary, just through fighting you may give them *more* meaning. Then they become more important. And this is happening. Those who fight with any desire, that desire becomes the center of their minds. If you fight sex, sex becomes the center. Then you are continuously engaged in it, occupied with it; it becomes like a wound. And wherever you look, that wound immediately projects itself, and whatever you see becomes sexual.

Mind has a mechanism, an old survival mechanism of fight or flight. Two are the ways of the mind: Either you can fight with something, or you can escape from it. If you are strong, then you fight. If you are weak, then you take flight; then you simply escape. But in both ways the "other" is important, the "other" is the center. You can fight, or you can escape from the world—from the world where desires are possible. You can go to the Himalayas. That, too, is a fight—the fight of the weak.

I have heard:

Once Mulla Nasruddin was shopping in a village. He left his donkey on the street and went into a shop to purchase something. When he came out, what he saw made him furious. Someone had painted his donkey completely red, bright red. So he was furious, and he shouted, "Who has done this? I will kill that man!"

A small boy was standing there. He said, "The man who has done this has just gone inside the pub."

So Nasruddin rushed into the pub, angry, mad. He said, "Who has done this? Who the hell has painted my donkey?"

A very big man, very strong, stood, and he said, "I did. What about it?"

Nasruddin said, "Thank you, sir. You have done such a beautiful job. I just came to tell you that the first coat is dry."

If you are strong, then you are ready to fight. If you are weak, then you are ready to fly, to take flight. But in neither case are you becoming stronger. In both cases the other has become the center of your mind. These are the two attitudes, fight or flight, and both are wrong because through both the mind is strengthened.

Patanjali says there is a third possibility: Don't fight and don't escape, just be alert. Just be conscious. Whatsoever is the case, just be a witness. Conscious effort means, one, searching for the inner source of happiness and, two, witnessing the old pattern of habits. Not fighting it, just witnessing it.

The first state of* vairagya, *desirelessness—cessation from self-indulgence in the thirst for sensuous pleasures, with conscious effort.

"Conscious effort" is the key. Consciousness is needed and effort is also needed. And the effort should be *conscious* because there can be unconscious efforts. You can be trained in such a way that you can drop certain desires without knowing that you have dropped them.

For example, if you are born in a vegetarian home, you will be eating vegetarian food. Nonvegetarian food is simply out of the question. You never dropped it consciously; you have been brought up in such a way that unconsciously it has dropped by itself. But this is not going to give you any integrity; this is not going to give you some spiritual strength. Unless you do something consciously, it is not really gained.

Many societies have tried this for their children—to bring them up in such a way that certain wrong things simply don't enter in their lives. They don't, but nothing is gained through it because the real thing to gain is consciousness. And consciousness can be gained through effort: If you are conditioned for something without effort, it is not a gain at all.

So in India there are many vegetarians—Jains, Brahmins, many people are vegetarians. Nothing is gained because it means nothing if you are vegetarian just by being born into a Jain family. It is not a conscious effort; you have not done anything about it. If you were born into a nonvegetarian family, you would have taken to nonvegetarian food similarly. Unless some conscious effort is made, your crystallization never happens. You have to do something on your own. When you do something on your own, you gain something.

Nothing is gained without consciousness, remember it. It is one of the ultimates. Nothing is gained without consciousness! You may become a perfect saint, but if you have not become saintly through consciousness it is futile, useless. You must struggle inch by inch, because in struggle more consciousness will be needed. The more consciousness you practice, the more conscious you become. And a moment comes when you become pure consciousness.

The first step is:

> ***Cessation from self-indulgence in the thirst for sensuous pleasures, with conscious effort.***

What to do? Whenever you are in any state of pleasure—sex, food, money, power, anything that gives you pleasure—meditate on it. Just try to find it: From where is it coming? Are you the source, or is the source somewhere else? If the source is somewhere else, then there is no possibility of any transformation because you will remain dependent on the source.

But fortunately the source is not anywhere else. It is within you. If you meditate, you will find it. It is knocking every moment from within: "I am here!" Once you have the feeling that it is knocking every moment, and you were creating only situations outside in which it was happening, then it can happen without those situations. Then you need not depend on anybody, on food, on sex, on power, anything. You are enough unto yourself. Once you have come to this feeling, the feeling of enoughness, then indulgence—the mind to indulge, the indulgent mind—disappears.

That doesn't mean you will not enjoy food. You will enjoy it more! But now food is not the source of your happiness, *you* are the source. You are not dependent on food, you are not addicted to it. That doesn't mean you will not enjoy sex. You can enjoy more, but now it is fun, play; it is just a celebration. You are not dependent on it, it is not the source.

And once two persons, two lovers can find this—that the other is not the source of their pleasure—they stop fighting with the other. They start loving the other for the first time.

> A person who holds the key of your happiness is your jailer. Lovers fight because they see that the other has the key: "He can make me happy or unhappy."

Otherwise you cannot love a person upon whom you are dependent in any way. You will hate him because he represents your dependence. Without him you cannot be happy, so he has the key. And a person who holds the key of your happiness is your jailer. Lovers fight because they see that the other has the key: "He can make me happy or unhappy."

Once you come to know that you are the source of your own happiness, and the other is the source of his own happiness . . . You can share your happiness, that's another thing, but you are not dependent. You can share, you can celebrate together. That's what love means: celebrating together, sharing together, not deriving happiness from each other, not exploiting each other. Exploitation cannot be love. Then you are using the other as a means, and whomever you use as a means will hate you. Lovers hate each other because they are using and exploiting each other, and love—which should be the deepest ecstasy—becomes the ugliest hell.

But once you know that you are the source of your happiness, that no one else is the source, you can share it freely. Then the other is not your enemy—not even an intimate enemy. For the first time friendship arises.

You can enjoy anything, and you will be able to enjoy only

when you are free. Only an independent person can enjoy. A person who is mad and obsessed with food cannot enjoy. He may fill his belly, but he cannot enjoy. His eating is violent. It is a sort of killing—he is killing the food; he is destroying the food. And lovers who feel that their happiness depends on the other are fighting, trying to dominate the other. They are trying to kill the other, to destroy the other.

You will be able to enjoy everything more when you know that the source is within. Then the whole of life becomes a play, and moment to moment you can go on celebrating, infinitely.

This is the first step, with effort. With consciousness and effort, you achieve desirelessness. Patanjali says this is the first because even effort, even consciousness, is not good because it means that some struggle, some hidden struggle is still happening.

The second and last step of *vairagya,* the last state of desirelessness:

> *Cessation of all desiring by knowing the innermost nature of* **purusha,** *the supreme self.*

First you have to know that you are the source of all happiness that happens to you; second, you have to know the total nature of your inner self. First you are the source; second, what is this source? First, just this much is enough—that you are the source of your happiness. And second, what this source is in its totality, this *purusha,* inner self, is to know "Who am I?" in its totality.

Once you know this source in its totality, you have known all. Then the whole universe is within—not only happiness. Then all that exists, exists within—not only happiness. Then God is not somewhere sitting in the clouds, he exists within. Then *you* are the source, the root source of all. Then *you* are the center.

And once you become the center of existence, once you know that you are the center of existence, all misery disappears. Now desirelessness becomes spontaneous, *sahaj.* No effort, no striving, no maintaining is needed. *It is so.* It has become natural. You are not pulling it or pushing it. Now there is no "I" who can pull and push.

Remember this: Struggle creates the ego. If you struggle in the world, it creates a gross ego: "I am someone with money, with prestige, with power." If you struggle within, it creates a subtle ego: "I am pure; I am a saint; I am a sage." But the "I" remains with struggle. So there are pious egoists who have a very subtle ego. They may not be worldly people—they are not; they are otherworldly—but struggle is there. They have "achieved" something. That achievement still carries the last shadow of "I."

The second step and the final step of desirelessness, for Patanjali, is total disappearance of the ego. Just nature flowing—no "I," no conscious effort. That doesn't mean you will not be conscious; you will be perfect consciousness—but with no effort implied to be conscious. There will be no *self*-consciousness, only pure consciousness. You have accepted yourself and existence as it is.

A total acceptance—this is what Lao Tzu calls Tao, the river flowing toward the sea. It is not making any effort; it is not in any hurry to reach the sea. Even if it doesn't reach, it will not get frustrated. Even if it reaches in millions of years, everything is OK. The river is simply flowing because flowing is its nature. No effort is there. It will go on flowing.

When desires for the first time are noted and observed, effort arises—a subtle effort. Even the first step is a subtle effort. You start trying to be aware: "From where is my happiness coming?" You have to do something, and that doing will create the ego. That's why Patanjali says this is only the beginning, and you must remember that it is not the end. In the end, not only have desires disappeared, *you* also have disappeared. Only the inner being has remained in its flow.

This spontaneous flow is the supreme ecstasy because no misery is possible for it. Misery comes through expectation, demand. There is no one to expect, to demand—so whatever happens, it is good. Whatever happens, it is a blessing. You cannot compare with anything else; *it is the case.* And because there is no comparing with the past and with the future—there is no one to compare—you cannot perceive anything as misery, as pain. Even if pain happens in that situation, it will not be painful. Try to understand this. This is difficult.

Jesus is being crucified. Christians have painted Jesus as being very sad. They have even said that he never laughed, and in their churches they have the sad figure of Jesus everywhere. This is human; we can understand it because a person who is being crucified must be sad. He must be in inner agony; he must be in suffering. So Christians go on saying that Jesus suffered for our sins—he *suffered.* But this is absolutely wrong! If you ask Patanjali or me, this is absolutely wrong. Jesus cannot suffer; it is impossible for Jesus to suffer. And if he suffers, then there is no difference between you and him. Pain is there, but he cannot suffer.

This may look mysterious, but it is not; this is simple. Pain is there—as far as we can see from the outside, Jesus is being crucified, insulted. His body is being destroyed. Pain is there, but Jesus cannot suffer. Because in this moment when Jesus is crucified, he cannot ask. He has no demand. He cannot say, "This is wrong. This should not be so. I should be crowned, and I am crucified."

If he has this in this mind—that "I should be crowned, and I am crucified"—then there will be pain. If he has no future orientation in the mind other than "I should be crowned," no expectation for the future, no fixed goal to reach, then wherever he has found himself is the goal. He cannot compare. This cannot be otherwise; this is the present moment that has been brought to him. This crucifixion *is* the crown.

And he cannot suffer because suffering means resistance. You have to resist something; only then you can suffer. Try it—it will be difficult for you to be crucified, but there are small daily crucifixions. They will do. You have a pain in the leg, or you have a headache. You may not have observed the mechanism of it—you have a headache, and you constantly struggle and resist. You don't want it, you are against it. You divide things—you are somewhere standing within the head, and the headache is there. You and the headache are separate, and you insist that it should not be so. This is the real problem.

> When there is no one to resist, even a headache is not painful. The fight creates the pain. The pain means always fighting against the pain—that's the real pain.

Just once try not to fight. Flow with the headache; become the headache. And say, "This is the case. This is how my head is at this moment, and at this moment nothing is possible. It may go away in the future, but in this moment the headache is there." Don't resist. Allow it to happen, become one with it. Don't pull yourself separate, flow into it. And then there will be a sudden upsurge of a new type of happiness you have not known. When there is no one to resist, even a headache is not painful. The fight creates the pain. The pain means always fighting against the pain—that's the real pain.

Jesus accepts. This is how his life has come—to the cross, this is the destiny. This is what in the East they have always called fate, *bhagya,* kismet. So there is no point in arguing with your fate, there is no point in fighting it. You cannot do anything; it is happening. Only one thing is possible for you: You can flow with it, or you can fight with it. If you fight, it becomes more agony. If you flow with it, the agony is less. And if you can flow totally, agony disappears. You have become the flow.

Try it when you have a headache, try it when you have an ill body, try it when you have some pain—just flow with it. And once you do, if you can allow, you will have come to one of the deepest secrets of life: that pain disappears if you flow with it. And if you can flow totally, pain becomes happiness.

But this is not something logical to be understood. You can comprehend it intellectually, but that won't do. Try it existentially. There are everyday situations. Every moment something is wrong—flow with it, and see how you transform the whole situation, and through that transformation you transcend it.

A Buddha can never be in pain; that is impossible. Only an ego can be in pain. Ego is a must in order to be in pain. And if the ego is there, you can also transform your pleasures into pain; if the ego is not there you can transform your pains into pleasures. The secret lies with the ego.

The last state of* vairagya, *desirelessness: cessation of all desiring by knowing the innermost nature of* purusha, *the supreme self.

How does it happen? Just by knowing the innermost core of yourself, the *purusha,* the dweller within. Just by knowing it! Patanjali says, Buddha says, Lao Tzu says the same: Just by knowing it, all desires disappear.

This is mysterious, and the logical mind is bound to ask how it can happen that just by knowing them, all desires disappear. It happens because now, not knowing themselves, all desires have arisen. Desires are simply the ignorance of the self. Why? All that you are seeking through desires is there, hidden in the self. If you know the self, desires will disappear.

For example, you are asking for power—everybody is asking for power. Power creates madness in everybody. It seems to be just that human society has existed in such a way that everybody is power addicted.

The child is born helpless—this is the first feeling that you all carry with you, always. The child is born, he is helpless, and a helpless child wants power. That's natural because everybody is more powerful than he is. The mother is powerful, the father is powerful, the brothers are powerful; everybody is powerful, and the child is absolutely helpless. Of course, the first desire that arises is to have power—to know how to grow powerful, how to be dominating. And the child starts being political from that very moment. He starts learning tricks of how to dominate. If he cries too much, he comes to know that he can dominate through crying. He can dominate the whole house just by crying. So he learns crying. And women continue it even when they are not children; they have learned the secret, and they continue it. And they have to continue it because they remain helpless. That's power politics.

The child knows a trick, and he can create disturbance. He can create such a disturbance that you have to accept and compromise with him. And every moment he feels deeply that the only thing that is needed is power, more power. He will learn, he will go to school, he will grow, he will love, but behind everything—his education, love, play—he will be finding out how to get more power. Through education he will want to dominate, to come first in the class so he can be dominating, to learn how to get more money so he can be dominating, to learn how to go on growing the influence and the territory of domination. The whole of his life he will be after power.

Many lives are simply wasted. And even if you get power, what are you going to do? Simply, a childish wish is fulfilled. So when you become a Napoleon or a Hitler, suddenly you become aware that the whole effort has been useless, futile. Just a childish wish has been fulfilled, that's all. Now what to do? What to do with this power? If the wish is fulfilled, you are frustrated; if the wish is not fulfilled, you are frustrated. And it cannot be fulfilled absolutely because no one can be so powerful that he can feel "Now it is enough"—no one! The world is so complex that even a Hitler feels powerless in moments, even a Napoleon feels powerless in moments. Nobody can feel absolutely powerful, and nothing can satisfy you.

When one comes to know one's self, one comes to know the source of absolute power. Then the desire for power disappears—because you were already a king, and you were only thinking that you were a beggar.

But when one comes to know one's self, one comes to know the source of absolute power. Then the desire for power disappears—because you were already a king, and you were only thinking that you were a beggar. You were struggling to be a bigger beggar, a greater beggar, and you were already the king! Suddenly you come to realize that you don't lack anything. You are not helpless; you are the source of all energies, you are the very source of life. That childhood feeling of powerlessness was created by others. And it is a vicious circle they created in you because it was created in them by their parents and so on and so forth.

Your parents are creating the feeling in you that you are powerless. Why? Because only through this can they feel that *they* are powerful. You may think that you love your children very much—but that doesn't seem to be the case. You love power, and when you get children, when you become mothers and fathers, you are powerful. Nobody else may be listening to you; you may be nothing in the world, but at least within the boundaries of your home you are powerful. You can at least torture small children.

And look at fathers and mothers: They *do* torture their children! And they torture in such a loving way that you cannot even say to them, "You are torturing." They are torturing the children "for their own good." For the children's own good! They are "helping them to grow." They feel powerful. Psychologists say that many people go into the teaching profession just to feel powerful because with thirty children at your disposal you are a king.

It is reported that one king named Aurangajeb was imprisoned by his son. When he was imprisoned, he wrote a letter and he said, "Only one wish—if you can fulfill it, it will be good, and I will be very happy. Just send thirty children to me so that I can teach them in my imprisonment."

The son is reported to have said, "My father has always remained a king, and he cannot lose his kingdom. So even in the prison he needs thirty children so he can teach them."

Look! Go into a school! The teacher sitting on his chair—he has absolute power, just the master of everything that is happening there. People want children not because they love—because if they love, really, the world will be totally different. If you love your child, the world will be totally different. You will not do anything to make him feel helpless; you will give him so much love that he will feel that he is powerful. If you give love, then he will never be asking for power. He will not become a political leader; he will not run for election. He will not try to accumulate money and go mad after it. Because he knows it is useless—he is already powerful; love is enough.

But when nobody is giving love, then the child will create substitutes. All your desires, whether for power, for money or prestige, all show that something was taught to you in your childhood, something has been conditioned in your biocomputer, and you are following that conditioning without looking inside to see if whatsoever you are asking for is already there.

> Something was taught to you in your childhood, something has been conditioned in your biocomputer, and you are following that conditioning without looking inside to see if what you are asking for is already there.

Patanjali's whole effort is to silence your biocomputer so that it doesn't interfere. This is what meditation is. It is putting your biocomputer, for certain moments, into silence, into a non-chattering state so that you can look within and hear your deepest nature. Just a glimpse will change you because then this biocomputer cannot deceive you. This biocomputer goes on saying that, "Do this . . . do that." It goes on continuously manipulating you: "You must have more power; otherwise you are nobody."

If you look within, there is no need to be anybody. There is no need to be "somebody." You are already accepted as you are. The whole existence accepts you, is happy about you. You are a flowering—an individual flowering different from any other, unique, and existence welcomes you; otherwise you could not be here. You are here only because you are accepted. You are here only because God loves you or the universe loves you or existence needs you. You are needed.

Once you know your innermost nature—what Patanjali calls the *purusha* . . . the *purusha* means the inner dweller. The body is just a house; the inner dweller, the indwelling consciousness, is *purusha.* Once you know this indwelling consciousness, nothing else is needed. You are enough, more than enough. You are perfect as you are. You are absolutely accepted, welcomed. Existence becomes a blessing. Desires disappear. They were part of self-ignorance. With self-knowledge they disappear, they evaporate.

Abhyasa, constant inner practice—conscious effort to be more and more alert, to be more and more a master of oneself, to be less and less dominated by habits, by mechanical, robotlike mechanisms—and *vairagya,* desirelessness. With these two attained, one becomes a yogi; with these two attained, one has attained the goal.

> Find out what it is that gives you happiness, from where it comes, and move in that direction. Desires, by and by, go on disappearing.

I will repeat: But don't create a fight. Allow all this happening to be more and more spontaneous. Don't fight with the negative;

rather, create the positive. Don't fight with sex, with food, with anything. Rather, find out what it is that gives you happiness, from where it comes, and move in that direction. Desires, by and by, go on disappearing.

And second: Be more and more conscious. Whatsoever is happening, be more and more conscious. And remain in that moment, and accept that moment. Don't ask for something else. You will not be creating misery then. If pain is there, let it be there. Remain in it, and flow in it. The only condition is, remain alert. Knowingly, watchfully move into it. Flow into it; don't resist.

When pain disappears, the desire for pleasure also disappears. When you are not in anguish, you don't ask for indulgence. When anguish is not there, indulgence becomes meaningless. More and more you go on falling into the inner abyss. And it is so blissful, it is such a deep ecstasy that with even a glimpse of it, the whole world becomes meaningless. Then all that this world can give to you is of no use.

And this should not become a fighting attitude—you should not become a warrior, you should become a meditator. If you are meditating, things will spontaneously happen to you that will go on transforming and changing you. Start fighting and you have started suppressing, and suppression will lead you into more and more misery.

And you cannot deceive anybody. There are many people who are not only deceiving others, they go on deceiving themselves. They think they are not in misery. They go on saying that they are not in misery, but their whole existence is miserable. When they are saying that they are not in misery, their faces, their eyes, their heart, everything is in misery.

I will tell you one anecdote and then finish.

I have heard that once it happened that twelve ladies reached purgatory. The officiating angel asked them, "Were any of you unfaithful to your husbands while on earth? If someone was unfaithful to her husband, she should raise her hand."

Blushingly, hesitating, by and by eleven ladies raised their hands.

The officiating angel took his phone, and spoke into it: "Hello! Is that hell? Have you got room for twelve unfaithful wives? And one of them is stone deaf!"

It doesn't matter whether you say or not—your face, your very being, shows everything. You may say you are not miserable, but the way you say it, the way you are, shows that you are miserable. You cannot deceive anybody, and there is no point to that—because no one can deceive anybody else, you can only deceive yourself.

Remember, if you are miserable you have created all of this. Let it penetrate deep in your heart that you have created your sufferings because this is going to be the formula, the key. If you have created your sufferings, only then can you destroy them. If someone else has created them, you are helpless. You have created your miseries, and you can destroy them. You have created them through wrong habits, wrong attitudes, addictions, desires.

Drop this pattern, look afresh. And this very life is the ultimate joy that is possible to human consciousness.

4

THE EIGHT STEPS

By practicing the different steps of yoga for the destruction of impurity, there arises spiritual illumination that develops into awareness of reality. The eight steps of yoga are: self-restraint, fixed observance, posture, breath regulation, abstraction, concentration, contemplation, and trance.

THE light that you seek is within you, so the search is going to be an inward search. It is not a journey to some goal in outer space; it is a journey into the inner space. You have to reach your core—that which you are seeking is already within you; you just have to peel the onion. Layers and layers of ignorance are there; the diamond is hidden in the mud. The diamond doesn't have to be created, the diamond is already there—only the layers of mud have to be removed.

This is very basic to understand: The treasure is already there. Maybe you don't have the key—the key has to be found but not the treasure. This is basic and very radical because the whole effort will depend on this understanding. If the treasure has to be created, then it is going to be a very long process, and nobody can be certain whether it can be created or not.

Only the key has to be found. The treasure is there, just nearby. A few layers of blocks have to be removed.

That's why the search for truth is negative. It is not a positive search. You don't have to add something to your being; rather, you have to delete something. You have to cut something away from you. The search for truth is surgical. It is not medical, it is surgical. Nothing is to be added to you; on the contrary, something has to be removed, negated. Hence the method of the *Upanishads: Neti, neti;* neither this nor that. The meaning of *neti, neti* is to go on negating until you reach to the negator; go on negating until there is not any possibility to negate; only you are left, you in your core, in your consciousness, which cannot be negated—because who will negate it? So go on negating: "I am neither this nor that." Go on—*"Neti, neti"*—and then a point comes when only you are, the negator. There is nothing else to cut anymore. The surgery is over; you have come to the treasure.

The search for truth is surgical. It is not medical, it is surgical. Nothing is to be added to you; on the contrary, something has to be removed, negated.

If this is understood rightly, then the burden is not very heavy. The search is very light; you can move easily, knowing well all the time on the way that the treasure may be forgotten, but it is not lost. You may not be able to know exactly where it is, but it is within you. You can rest assured, there is no uncertainty about it. In fact, even if you want to lose it, you cannot lose it because it is your very being. It is not something external to you; it is intrinsic.

People come to me and say, "We are in search of God." I ask them, "Where have you lost him? Why are you seeking? Have you lost him somewhere? If you have lost him somewhere, then tell me where you have lost him because only there will you be able to find him."

They say, "No, we have not lost him. . . ." Then why are you seeking? Then just close your eyes. Maybe because of the search you cannot find him. Maybe you are too concerned with seeking. You have not looked at your own inner being to see that the king of kings is sitting there already, waiting for you to come home. And you are a great seeker, so you are going to Mecca and Medina, Kashi and Kailash. You are a great seeker. You are going all over the world, except one place: where you are! The seeker is the sought.

When one is quiet and still, nothing new is achieved; one simply starts understanding that looking outside was the whole reason for missing. Looking in, it is there. It has always been there. There has never been a single moment when it was not there, and there will never be a single moment when it will not be there—because God is not external, truth is not external to you. It is you glorified; it is you in your total splendor; it is you in your absolute purity. If you understand this, then these sutras of Patanjali will be very simple.

> ***By practicing the different steps of yoga for the destruction of impurity, there arises spiritual illumination that develops into awareness of reality.***

He is not saying that something is to be created; he is saying something is to be destroyed. You are already *more* than your being—this is the problem. You have gathered too much around you; the diamond has gathered too much mud. The mud has to be washed away, and suddenly there is the diamond.

"By practicing the different steps of yoga for the destruction of impurity . . ." It is not a creation of purity or holiness or divineness, it is just a destruction of impurity. Pure you are.

Holy you are. The whole path becomes totally different. Then a few things have to be cut and dropped; a few things have to be eliminated.

Deep down this is the meaning of *sannyas,* renunciation. It is not to renounce the house, not to renounce the family, not to renounce the children—that looks so cruel; how can a man of compassion do it? It is not to renounce the wife because that is not the problem at all. The wife is not obstructing God, and neither are the children creating barriers, nor is the house. No, if you renounce them, you have not understood. Renounce something else that you have been gathering within yourself.

If you want to renounce the house, renounce the real house—that is, the body in which you live and reside. And by renouncing I don't mean go and commit suicide because that won't be renouncing. Just knowing that you are not the body is enough; there is no need to be cruel to the body, either. You may not be the body, but the body is also godly. You may not be the body, but the body is alive on its own. It also partakes of life; it is part of this totality. Don't be cruel to it, don't be violent to it. Don't be a masochist. Religious people almost always become masochists. Or they were already masochistic, and religion becomes a rationalization, and they start torturing themselves.

You may not be the body, but the body is also godly. Don't be cruel to it, don't be violent to it. Don't be a masochist.

Don't be a self-torturer. There are two types of torturers and violent people: One type is the sadists who torture others—the politicians, the Adolf Hitlers. And then there are self-torturers the masochists, who torture themselves—the so-called religious people, saints, mahatmas. They are the same, the violence is the same. Whether you torture anyone else's body or your own makes no difference—you torture all the same.

Renunciation is not self-torture. If it is self-torture, it is only politics standing on its head. It may be that you are so cowardly that you cannot manage to torture others, so you can torture only your own body. Ninety-nine out of a hundred so-called religious people are self-torturers, cowards. They wanted to torture others, but there was fear and danger, and they couldn't do it. So they have found a very innocent victim, vulnerable, helpless: their own body. And they torture it in millions of ways.

No, renunciation means knowledge; renunciation means awareness; renunciation means realization—realization of the fact that you are not the body. It is finished. You live in it knowing well that you are not it. When you are unidentified with it, the body is beautiful; it is one of the greatest mysteries in existence. It is the very temple where the king of kings is hiding.

When you understand what renunciation is, you understand that this is *neti, neti.* You say, "I am not this body because I am aware of the body; the very awareness makes me separate and different." Go deeper. Go on peeling the onion: "I am not the thoughts because they come and go, but I remain. I am not the emotions. . . ." They come—sometimes very strong, and you forget yourself completely in them—but then they go. There was a time that they were not, and *you* were; there was a time that *they* were, and you were hidden in them. There is again a time when they have gone, and you are sitting there. You cannot be the emotions; you are separate from them.

Go on peeling the onion: No, you are not the body. Thinking

you are not, feeling you are not. And if you know that you are not these three layers, your ego simply disappears without leaving a trace behind—because your ego is nothing but identification with these three layers.

Then you *are,* but you cannot say "I." The word loses meaning. The ego is not there; you have come home.

This is the meaning of *sannyas*: It is negating all that you are not but are identified with. This is the surgery. This is the destruction.

> ***By practicing the different steps of yoga for the destruction of impurity . . .***

And this is impurity: Thinking yourself to be that which you are not is the impurity. Don't misunderstand me because there is always a possibility that you might misunderstand that the body is impure. I am not saying that. You can have pure water in one container and pure milk in another. Mix them together—the mixture is not now doubly pure. Both were pure: The water was pure, pure water from the Ganges, and the milk was pure. Now you mix two purities, and one impurity is born—not that the purity is doubled. What has happened? Why do you call this mixture of water and milk impure? Impurity means the entering of a foreign element, that which does not belong to it, is not natural to it—is an intruder that has trespassed into its territory. It is not only that the milk is impure, the water is also impure. Two purities meet and become impure.

So when I say renounce the impurities, I don't mean that your body is impure. I don't mean that your mind is impure. I don't even mean that your feelings are impure. Nothing is impure—but when you get identified, *in that identification is impurity.*

Everything is pure. Your body is perfect if it functions on its own, and you don't interfere. Your consciousness is pure if it functions on its own, and the body does not interfere. If you live in a noninterfering existence, you are pure.

> Your body is perfect if it functions on its own, and you don't interfere. Your consciousness is pure if it functions on its own, and the body does not interfere. If you live in a noninterfering existence, you are pure.

Everything is pure. I'm not condemning the body. I never condemn anything. Make it a point to always remember. I am not a condemner. Everything is beautiful as it is. But identification creates the impurity.

When you start thinking you are the body, you have intruded upon the body. And when you intrude upon the body, the body immediately reacts and intrudes upon you. Then there is impurity.

Says Patanjali:

> ***By practicing the different steps of yoga for the destruction of impurity . . .***

For the destruction of identity, identification, for the destruction of the mess that you are in—the chaos, where everything has become everything else . . . Nothing is clear, no center is functioning on its own; you have become a crowd. Everything goes on interfering into everything else's nature. This is impurity.

> ***. . . for the destruction of impurity, there arises a spiritual illumination.***

And once the impurity is destroyed, suddenly there is illumination. It doesn't come from outside, it is your innermost being in its purity, in its innocence, in its virginity. A luminosity arises in you; everything is clear. With the crowds of confusion gone, the clarity of perception arises. Now you can see everything as it is. There are no projections; there is no imagination; there is no perversion of any reality. You simply see things as they are. Your eyes are vacant; your being is silent. Now you don't have anything in you, so you cannot project. You become a passive onlooker, a witness, a *sakshin*—and that is the purity of being.

> ***. . . there arises spiritual illumination that develops into awareness of reality.***

Then, the eight steps of yoga. Follow me very slowly, because here is the central teaching of Patanjali:

> ***The eight steps of yoga are self-restraint, fixed observance, posture, breath regulation, abstraction, concentration, contemplation, and trance.***

The eight steps of yoga—this is the whole science of yoga in one sentence, in one seed. Many things are implied. First, let me tell you the exact meaning of each step. And remember, Patanjali calls them "steps" and "limbs" both. They are both. They are steps because one has to be followed by another; there is a sequence of growth. But they are not only steps, they are also limbs of the body of yoga. They have an internal unity, an organic unity; that is the meaning of calling them limbs.

For example, my hands, my feet, my heart—they don't function separately. They are not separate; they are an organic unity.

If the heart stops, then the hand will not move. Everything is joined together. They are not just like steps on a ladder because every rung on the ladder is separate; if one rung is broken, the whole ladder is not broken. So Patanjali says they are steps because they have a certain sequential growth—but they are also *angas,* limbs of a body, organic. You cannot drop any of them. Steps can be dropped; limbs cannot be dropped. You can make two steps in one jump, you can drop one step, but limbs cannot be dropped; they are not mechanical parts. You cannot remove them. They make up you. They belong to the whole; they are not separate. The whole functions through them as a harmonious unit.

So these eight limbs of yoga are both: steps in the sense that each follows the other—and they are in a deep relationship. The second cannot come before the first—the first has to be first, and the second has to be second, and the eighth will come to be the eighth. It cannot be the fourth, it cannot be the first. So they are steps, and they are also an organic unity—limbs.

Yam means self-restraint. In English the word becomes a little different. Not just a little different, really; the whole meaning of *yam* is lost—because in English, self-restraint looks like suppressing, repressing. And after Freud, these two words *suppression* and *repression* have become four-letter words, ugly.

Self-restraint is not repression. In the days when Patanjali used the word *yam,* it had a totally different meaning. Words go on changing. Even now, in India, too, *samyam,* which comes from *yam,* means control, repression. The meaning is lost.

You may have heard an anecdote. It is said about King George I of England that he went to see St. John's Cathedral when it was built. It was a masterpiece of art. The builder, the architect, the artist was present; his name was Christopher Wren. The king looked at him and complimented him. He said three things: "It is amusing. It is awful. It is artificial." Christopher Wren was so delighted with the compliments . . . but you are no doubt surprised. Those words don't have the same meaning anymore. In those days, more than three hundred years ago, "amusing" meant amazing, "awful" meant awe-inspiring, and "artificial" meant artistic.

Each word has a biography, and it changes many times. As life changes, everything changes. Words take on new colors. And, in fact, only the words that have the capacity to change remain alive; otherwise they go dead. Orthodox words, reluctant to change—they die. Alive words, with the capacity to collect a new meaning around them, only they live. And they live in many, many meanings for centuries.

Yam was a beautiful word in Patanjali's day, one of the most beautiful. After Freud, the word has become ugly—not only the meaning has changed but the whole flavor, the whole taste of the word.

Self-restraint does not mean to repress oneself. It simply means to direct one's life—not to repress the energies but to direct them, to give them a direction.

To Patanjali, self-restraint does not mean to repress oneself. It simply means to direct one's life—not to repress the energies but to direct them, to give them a direction. Because you can live a life that goes on moving in opposite directions, in many directions, and then you will never reach anywhere. It is just like a car: The driver goes a few miles to the north, then changes his mind; goes a few miles to the south, then changes his mind; then goes a few miles to the west, then changes his mind—and he goes on this way. He will die where he was born! He will never reach anywhere, he will never have the feeling of fulfillment.

You can go on moving in many ways, but unless you have a direction, you are moving uselessly. You will feel more and more frustrated and nothing else.

To create self-restraint means first to give a direction to your life energy. Life energy is limited; if you go on using it in absurd, undirected ways, you will not reach anywhere. You will be emptied of the energy sooner or later—and that emptiness will not be the emptiness of a Buddha; it will be simply a negative emptiness. Nothing inside, an empty container; you will be dead before you are dead.

But these limited energies that have been given to you by nature, existence, God, or whatsoever you like to call it—these limited energies can be used in such a way that they can become the door for the unlimited. If you move rightly, if you move consciously, if you move alertly, gathering all your energies and moving in one direction, if you are not a crowd but become an individual—that is the meaning of *yam*.

Ordinarily you are a crowd, many voices inside. One says, "Go to this direction." Another says, "That is useless. Go this way." One says, "Go to the temple." And yet another says, "The theater will be better." And you are never at ease anywhere because wherever you are, you will be repenting. If you go to the theater, the voice that was in favor of the temple will go on creating trouble for you: "What are you doing here wasting your time? You could have been in the temple—and prayer is beautiful. And nobody knows what is happening there—nobody knows, this may have been the opportunity for your enlightenment, and you have missed it." If you go to the temple, it will be the same; the voice that was insisting to go to the theater will go on saying, "What are you doing here? Like a foolish man you are sitting here, and you have prayed before and nothing happens—why are you wasting your time?" And all around you, you will see fools sitting and doing useless things, and nothing happens. In the theater, who knows what excitement, what ecstasy was possible? You are missing.

If you are not an individual, a unitary being, then wherever you are, you will always be missing. You will never be at home anywhere; you will always be going somewhere or other and never arriving anywhere. You will become mad! The life that is against *yam* will become mad. It is not surprising that in the West more mad people exist than in the East. The East—knowingly or unknowingly—still follows a life of a little self-restraint. In the West, to think about self-restraint looks like becoming a slave; to be against self-restraint looks like you are free, independent.

But unless you are an individual, you cannot be free. Your freedom will be a deception; it will be nothing but suicide. You will kill yourself, destroy your possibilities, your energies. And one day you will feel that for your whole life you tried so much, but nothing has been gained, no growth has come out of it.

Self-restraint means—the first meaning—to give a direction to life. Self-restraint means to become a little more centered.

How can you become a little more centered? Once you give a direction to your life, immediately a center, starts happening within you. Direction creates the center, and then the center gives direction. And they are mutually fulfilling.

Unless you are self-restrained, the second is not possible—that's why Patanjali calls them "steps."

* * *

The second step is *niyam,* fixed observance—a life that has a discipline, a life that has a regularity about it, a life that is lived in a very disciplined way, not hectic. Regularity . . . but that, too, will sound to you like slavery. All the beautiful words of Patanjali's time have become ugly now. But I tell you: Unless you have a regularity in your life, a discipline, you will be a slave of your instincts. And you may think this is freedom, but you will be a slave of all the vagrant thoughts—that is not freedom. You may not have any visible master, but you will have many invisible masters within you, and they will go on dominating you. Only a man who has a regularity about him can become the master someday.

That, too, is far away still because the real master happens only when the eighth step is achieved—that is the goal. Then a man becomes a *jina,* a conqueror. Then a man becomes a Buddha, one who is awakened. Then a man becomes a Christ, a savior, because if you are saved, suddenly you become a savior for others. Not that you try to save them; just your presence is a saving influence. The second is *niyam,* fixed observance.

The third step is posture. And every step comes out of the first, the preceding one: When you have regularity in life, only then can you attain to posture, *asan.* Try *asan* sometimes; just try to sit silently. You cannot sit—the body tries to revolt against you. Suddenly you start feeling pain here and there, the legs are going dead; suddenly you feel in many spots of the body a restlessness. You had never felt it before—why is it that just by sitting silently so many problems arise? You feel ants are crawling on you. Look and you will see that there are no ants; the body is deceiving you.

The body is not ready to be disciplined. The body is spoiled;

the body does not want to listen to you. It has become its own master, and you have always followed it. Now, even to sit silently for a few minutes has become almost impossible. People pass through such hell if you tell them to just sit silently. If I say this to somebody, he says, "Just sit silently, not doing anything?"—as if "doing" is an obsession. He says, "At least give me a mantra so I can go on chanting inside." He needs some occupation; just sitting silently seems to be difficult.

And that is the most beautiful possibility that can happen to a person: just sitting silently doing nothing.

Asan means a relaxed posture. You are so relaxed in it, you are so restful in it that there is no need to move the body at all. In that moment, suddenly, you transcend the body.

The body is trying to bring you down when it says, "Now, look, many ants are crawling on you." Or you suddenly feel an urge to scratch, itching; the body is saying, "Don't go so far away. Come back. Where are you going?"—because the consciousness is moving upward, going far away from the bodily existence. The body starts revolting: "You have never done such a thing!" The body creates problems for you because once the problem is there, you will have to come back. The body is asking for your attention: "Give me your attention." It will create pain, it will create itching; you will feel like scratching. Suddenly the body is no longer ordinary, the body is in revolt. It is a "body politic."

Asan means a relaxed posture. You are so relaxed in it, you are so restful in it that there is no need to move the body at all. In that moment, suddenly, you transcend the body.

You are being called back: "Don't go so far away. Be occupied. Remain here, remain tethered to the body and to the earth." You are moving toward the sky, and the body feels afraid.

Asan comes only to a person who lives a life of restraint, fixed observance, regularity; then posture is possible. Then you can simply sit because the body knows that you are a disciplined person; if you want to sit, you will sit, and nothing can be done against you. The body can go on saying things . . . by and by it stops. Nobody is there to listen. It is not suppression; you are not suppressing the body. On the contrary, the body is trying to suppress you. It is not suppression; you are not telling the body to do anything, you are simply resting.

But the body does not know any rest because you have never given rest to it. You have always been restless. The very word *asan* means to be in deep rest. And if you can do that, many things will become possible to you.

If the body can be in rest, then you can regulate your breathing. You are moving deeper because breath is the bridge from the body to the soul, from the body to the mind. If you can regulate the breathing—that is, *pranayam*—you have power over your mind.

Have you ever noticed that whenever the mind changes, the rhythm of the breath immediately changes? If you do the opposite—if you change that rhythm of the breath—the mind has to change immediately. When you are angry, you cannot breathe silently, otherwise the anger will disappear. Try it. When you are feeling angry your breath goes chaotic, it becomes irregular, loses all-rhythm, becomes noisy, restless. It is no longer a harmony. A discord starts being there; the accord is lost. Try one thing: Whenever you are getting angry, just relax and let the breath be in rhythm. Suddenly you will feel the anger has disappeared. The anger cannot exist without a particular type of breathing in your body.

When you are making love, the breath changes, becomes very violent. When you are very much filled with sexuality, the breath changes. Sex has a little violence in it; lovers are known to bite each other, sometimes even harm each other. And if you see two persons making love, you will see that some sort of fighting is going on. There is a little violence in it, and both are breathing chaotically; their breathing is not in rhythm, not in unison.

In Tantra, where much has been done around sex and the transformation of sex, they have worked very much on the rhythm of the breath. Tantra developed many techniques of changing the rhythm of the breath. If two lovers, while making love, can remain in a rhythmic breathing, in unison, so that both have the same rhythm, there will be no ejaculation. They can make love for hours because ejaculation is possible only when the breath is not in rhythm; only then can the body throw the energy out. If the breath is in rhythm, the body absorbs the energy; it never throws it out. Then you can make love for hours, and you don't lose energy. On the contrary, you gain because if a woman loves a man and a man loves a woman, they help each other to be recharged—because they are opposite energies. When opposite energies meet and spark, they charge each other; otherwise energy is lost, and after the lovemaking you feel a little cheated, deceived—so much promise and nothing comes into your hands; the hands remain empty.

After *asan* comes breath regulation, *pranayam.* Watch for a few days, and just take note: When you become angry, what is the rhythm of your breathing—is the exhalation long or the inhalation long or are they the same? Or is the inhalation very small and the exhalation very long or the exhalation very small and the inhalation very long? Just watch the proportion of inhalation and exhalation. When you are sexually aroused, watch, take note. When sometimes sitting silently and looking at the sky in the night, everything is quiet around you, just take note of how your breath is going. When you are feeling filled with compassion, watch, note it down. When you are in a fighting mood, watch, note it down. Just make a chart of your own breathing, and then you will know much.

And *pranayam* is not something that can be taught to you. You have to discover it yourself because everybody has a different rhythm to his breathing. Everybody's breathing and its rhythm is as different as their thumbprints. Breathing is an individual phenomenon; that's why I never teach it. You have to discover your own rhythm. Your rhythm may not be a rhythm for somebody else or may even be harmful for somebody else. *Your* rhythm—you have to find it.

Everybody's breathing and its rhythm is as different as their thumbprints. Breathing is an individual phenomenon; that's why I never teach it. You have to discover your own rhythm.

And it is not difficult. There is no need to ask any expert. Just keep a chart for one month of all your moods and states. Then you know which is the rhythm where you feel most restful, relaxed, in a deep let-go; which is the rhythm where you feel quiet, calm, collected, cool; which is the rhythm when suddenly you feel blissful. Filled with something unknown, overflowing—you have so much in that moment, you can give to the whole world, and it will not be exhausted. Feel and watch the moment when you feel that you are one with the universe, when you feel the separateness is no longer there, when there is a bridge. When you feel one with the trees and the birds and the rivers and the rocks, and the ocean and the sand—watch. You will find that there are many rhythms of your breath, a great spectrum from the most violent, ugly, miserable hell type to the most silent heaven type.

And then, when you have discovered your rhythm, practice it—make it a part of your life. By and by it becomes unconscious; then you breathe only in that rhythm. And with that rhythm your life will be the life of a yogi. You will not be angry, you will not feel so sexual, you will not feel so filled with hatred. Suddenly you will feel a transmutation is happening to you.

Pranayam is one of the greatest discoveries that has ever happened to human consciousness. Compared to *pranayam,* going to the moon is nothing—it looks very exciting, but it is nothing because even if you reach the moon, what will you do there? Even if you reach the moon, you will remain the same. You will do the same nonsense that you are doing here.

Pranayam is an inner journey. And *pranayam* is the fourth of only eight steps. Half the journey is completed on *pranayam.* A man who has learned *pranayam,* not from a teacher—because that is a false thing; I don't approve of it—but by his own discovery and alertness, a man who has learned his rhythm of being has achieved half the goal already. *Pranayam* is one of the most significant discoveries.

And after *pranayam,* breath regulation, is *pratyahar,* abstraction. *Pratyahar* is the same as the "repentance" of Christians. "Repent" is, in fact, in Hebrew, "return"—not repent but return, coming back. The *toba* of Mohammedans is not "repenting." That, too, has become colored with the meaning of repentance, but *toba* is also returning, coming back. And *pratyahar*, too, is returning, coming back—coming in, turning in, returning home. *Pratyahar* is possible after *pranayam* because *pranayam* will give you the rhythm. Now you know the whole spectrum—you know in what rhythm you are nearest to home and in what rhythm you are farthest from yourself. Violent, sexual, angry, jealous, possessive—you will find you are far away from yourself. In compassion, in love, in prayer, in gratitude, you will find yourself nearer home. After *pranayam, pratyahar,* return, is possible. Now you know the way—you already know how to step back.

Then comes *dharana.* After *pratyahar,* when you have started coming back nearer home, coming nearer your innermost core, you are just at the gate of your own being. *Pratyahar* brings you near the gate; *pranayam* is the bridge from the out to the in. *Pratyahar,* returning, is the gate, and then is the possibility of *dharana,* concentration. Now you become capable of bringing your mind to one object. First you gave direction to your body; first you gave direction to your life energy—now you give direction to your consciousness. Now the consciousness cannot be allowed to go anywhere and everywhere. Now it has to be brought to a goal. This goal is concentration, *dharana*: You fix your consciousness on one point.

When consciousness is fixed on one point, thoughts cease because thoughts are possible only when your consciousness goes on wavering—from here to there, from there to somewhere else. When your consciousness is continuously jumping like a monkey, then there are many thoughts, and your whole mind is just filled with crowds, a marketplace. Now there is a possibility—after *pranayam,* after *pratyahar,* there is a possibility—you can concentrate on one point.

If you can concentrate on one point, then comes the possibility of *dhyan.* In concentration you bring your mind to one point. In *dhyan* you also drop that point. Now you are totally centered, "nowhere-going"—because if you are going anywhere it is always going out. Even a single thought in concentration is something outside you—the object exists; you are not alone; there are two. Even in concentration there are two: the object and you. After concentration the object has to be dropped.

All the temples lead you only up to concentration. They cannot lead you beyond because all the temples have an object in them: The image of God is an object to concentrate on. All the temples lead you only up to *dharana,* concentration. That's why the higher a religion goes, the temple and the images disappear. They have to disappear. The temple should be absolutely empty so that only you are there—nobody else, no object. Just pure subjectivity.

The higher a religion goes, the temple and the images disappear. They have to disappear. The temple should be absolutely empty so that only you are there—nobody else, no object. Just pure subjectivity.

Dhyan is pure subjectivity, contemplation—not contemplating "something" because if you are contemplating something, it is concentration. In English there are no better words. Concentration means something is there to concentrate upon. *Dhyan* is meditation: Nothing is there, everything has dropped, but you are in an intense state of awareness. The object has dropped, but the subject has not fallen into sleep. Deeply concentrated, without any object, centered—but still the feeling of "I" will persist. It will hover. The object has fallen, but the subject is still there. You still feel you are.

This is not ego. In Sanskrit we have two words, *ahankar* and *asmita. Ahankar* means "I am." And *asmita* means "am." Just "amness"—no ego exists; just the shadow is left. You still feel, somehow, that you are. It is not a thought because if it is a thought that "I am," it is an ego. In meditation the ego has disappeared completely; but an *amness,* a shadowlike phenomenon, just a feeling, hovers around you—just a mistlike thing that just in the morning hovers around you. In meditation it is morning. The sun has not risen yet; it is misty: *asmita, amness* is still there.

You can still fall back. A slight disturbance—somebody starts talking, and you listen—meditation has disappeared, and you have come back to concentration. If you not only listen, but you also have started thinking about it, even concentration has disappeared; you have come back to *pratyahar.* And if not only are you thinking, but you have also become identified with the thinking, *pratyahar* has disappeared; you have fallen to *pranayam.* And if the thought has taken so much possession of you that your breathing rhythm is lost, *pranayam* has disappeared; you have fallen to *asan.* But if the thought and the breathing are so much disturbed that the body starts shaking or becomes restless, *asan* has disappeared.

They are related.

One can fall from meditation. Meditation is the most dangerous point in the world because that is the highest point from where you can fall, and you can fall badly. In India we have a word, *yogabhrasta*: one who has fallen from yoga. This word is very, very strange. It appreciates and condemns together. When we say somebody is a yogi, it is a great appreciation. When we say somebody is *yogabhrasta,* it is also a condemnation: The person has fallen from yoga. This person had attained up to meditation somewhere in a past life and then fell down. From meditation the possibility of going back to the world is still there—because of *asmita,* because of *amness.* The seed is still alive. It can sprout any moment; so the journey is not over.

When *asmita* also disappears, when you no longer know that you are—of course, you are, but there is no reflection upon it, no "I am," or even amness—then *samadhi* happens—trance, ecstasy. *Samadhi* is going beyond; then one never comes back. *Samadhi* is a point of no return. From there, nobody falls. A person in *samadhi* is a god: we call Buddha a god, Mahavir a god. A man in *samadhi* is no longer of this world. He may be *in* this world, but he is no longer *of* this world. He doesn't belong to it; he is an outsider. He may physically be here, but his home is somewhere else. He may walk on this earth, but he no longer walks on the earth. It is said about the man of *samadhi* that he lives in the world, but the world does not live in him.

These are the eight steps and eight limbs together. Limbs because they are so interrelated and so organically related; steps because you have to pass through them one by one. You cannot start from just anywhere, you have to start from *yam.*

Now a few more things—because this is such a central phenomenon for Patanjali that you have to understand a few things more. *Yam* is a bridge between you and others; self-restraint means restraining your behavior. *Yam* is a phenomenon between you and others, you and the society. It is a more conscious behavior: You don't react unconsciously; you don't react like a mechanism, like a robot. You become more conscious; you become more alert. You react only when there is some absolute necessity; then, too, you try so that that reaction should be a response and not a reaction.

A response is different from a reaction. The first difference is that a reaction is automatic, and a response is conscious. Somebody insults you, immediately you react and you insult him; there has not been a single moment's gap to understand—it is reaction. A person of self-restraint will wait, listen to the insult, think about it.

Gurdjieff used to say that his whole life changed because when his grandfather was dying and Gurdjieff was just nine years of age, he called him and told him, "I am a poor man and I have nothing to give to you, but I would like to give something. The only thing that I have been carrying like a treasure is this—this was given to me by my own father. You are very young, but remember it. Someday you will understand, so just remember it. Right now I don't hope that you can understand, but if you don't forget, someday you will understand." And this is the thing he told to Gurdjieff: "If somebody insults you, answer him after twenty-four hours have passed."

It became a transformation because how can you react after twenty-four hours? Reaction needs immediacy. Gurdjieff says, "Somebody would insult me, or somebody would say something wrong, and I would have to say, 'I will come back tomorrow. Only after twenty-four hours am I allowed to answer. I have given a promise to my grandfather, and he is dead, and the promise cannot be taken back. But I will come.' "

That man would be taken aback. He would not be able to understand what was the matter. And Gurdjieff would think about it. The more he would think, the more useless it would look. Sometimes he would feel that the man was right, whatsoever he had said was true. Then Gurdjieff would go and thank the man: "You brought to light something of which I was unaware." Sometimes he would come to know that the man was absolutely wrong. And when the man is absolutely wrong, why bother? Nobody bothers about lies. When you feel hurt, there must be some truth in it; otherwise you don't feel hurt. Then, too, there is no point.

And he said, "It came to pass that many times I tried my grandfather's formula, and by and by anger disappeared"—and not only anger: By and by he became aware that the same technique can be used for other emotions. And everything disappeared. Gurdjieff was one of the highest peaks that has been attained in this age, a buddha. And the whole journey started with a very small step, the promise given to a dying old man. It changed his whole life.

Yam is the bridge between you and others: Live consciously; relate with people consciously. Then the second two, *niyam* and *asan*—they are concerned with your body. The third, *pranayam* is again a bridge. As the first, *yam,* is a bridge between you and others, the second two are a preparation for another bridge. Your body is made ready through *niyam* and *asan,* and then *pranayam* is the bridge between the body and the mind. Then *pratyahar* and *dharana* are the preparation of the mind. *Dhyan,* again, is a bridge between the mind and the soul. And *samadhi* is the attainment. They are interlinked, a chain; and this is your whole life.

Your relation with others has to be changed. How you relate has to be transformed. If you continue to relate with others in the same way as you have always been doing, there is no possibility to change—you have to change your relationship. Watch how you behave with your wife or with your friend or with your children. Change it. There are a thousand and one things to be changed in your relationship. That is *yam,* control—but control, not suppression. Through understanding comes control. Through ignorance one goes on forcing and suppressing. Always do everything with understanding, and you never harm yourself or anybody else.

Yam is to create a congenial environment around yourself. If you are inimical to everybody—fighting, hateful, angry—how can you move inward? All these things will not allow you to move. You will be so disturbed on the surface that the inner journey will not be possible. To create a congenial, friendly atmosphere around you is *yam.* When you relate with others beautifully, consciously, they don't create trouble for you in your inner journey. They become a help, they don't hinder you. If you love your child, then when you are meditating, he will not disturb you. He will say to others, "Keep quiet. Pop is meditating." But if you don't love your child, and you are simply angry, then when you are meditating, he will create all sorts of nuisances. He unconsciously wants to take revenge. If you love your wife deeply, she will be helpful; otherwise she won't allow you to pray, she won't allow you to meditate—you are going beyond her control.

This I see every day: The husband becomes a *sannyasin,* and the wife comes crying: "What have you done to our family? You have destroyed us." Then I know the husband has not loved the wife; otherwise she would have been happy. She would have celebrated that her husband has become meditative. But he has not loved her—now, not only has he not loved her, he is moving inward so there will be no possibility in the future, either, of any love coming from him.

If you love a person, the person is always helpful for your growth because he knows, or she knows, that the more you grow, the more you will be capable of love. They know the taste of love. And all meditations will help you to love more, to be more beautiful in every way. But this happens every day. Everybody is making an effort to control the other.

A man of *yam* controls himself, not others. To others he gives freedom. But you try to control the other and never yourself. A man of *yam* controls himself and gives freedom to others—he loves so much that he can give freedom, and he loves himself so much that he controls himself. This has to be understood: He loves himself so much that he cannot dissipate his energies; he has to give them a direction.

Then, *niyam* and *asan* are for the body. A regular life is very healthy for the body because the body is a mechanism. You confuse the body if you lead an irregular life. Today you have taken your food at one o'clock; tomorrow you take your food at eleven o'clock; day after tomorrow you take it at ten o'clock—you confuse the body. The body has an inner biological clock; it moves in a pattern. If you take your food every day at exactly the same time, the body is always in a situation where she understands what is happening. And she is ready for the happening—the juices are flowing in the stomach at the right moment. Otherwise whenever you want to take the food, you can take it, but the juices will not be flowing. And if you take the food and the juices are not flowing, then the food becomes cold; then the digestion is difficult. The juices must be ready to receive the food while it is hot; then immediately absorption starts. Food can be absorbed in six hours if the

A regular life is very healthy for the body because the body is a mechanism. You confuse the body if you lead an irregular life.

juices are ready, waiting. If the juices are not waiting, then it takes twelve to eighteen hours. Then you feel heavy, lethargic. Then the food gives you life but does not give you pure life. It feels like a weight on your chest; you somehow carry yourself, drag yourself. And food can become such pure energy—but a regular life is needed.

You go to sleep every day at ten o'clock. The body knows. Exactly at ten o'clock the body gives you an alarm. I'm not saying become obsessive so that when your mother is dying, you go to sleep at ten o'clock then, too. I'm not saying that. Because people can become obsessive. . . . Don't create an obsession.

There are many stories about Immanuel Kant. He became obsessive about regularity; it became a madness. He had a fixed routine—so fixed, second to second, that if a guest had come, he would look at the clock, and he would not even say anything to the guest because speaking would take time. He would jump into bed, cover himself with the blanket, and go to sleep—and the guest was sitting there! The servant would come and say, "Now go because that was his bedtime." The servant became so attuned to Kant that there was no need to say, "Your food is ready" and no need to say, "Now you go to sleep." Only the time had to be said. The servant would come in the room and say, "It is eleven o'clock, sir." There was no need to say anything else.

Kant was so regular that the servant became the dictator—he would always threaten, "I will leave if you don't raise my pay." Immediately the pay had to be raised because another servant, a new man, would disturb the whole routine. Once they tried—a new man came, but it was not possible because Kant was living second to second.

He would go to the university—he was a great teacher and a great philosopher. One day the road was muddy—it was raining—and one of his shoes got stuck in the mud. So he left it there; otherwise he would be late. He went the rest of the way with one shoe on. It was said in the university area of Konigsberg that people seeing him would set their watches because everything he did was absolutely punctual.

A new neighbor purchased the house adjacent to Kant's house, and he started planting new trees. Every day at exactly five o'clock in the evening, Kant used to come to that side of the house and sit near the window, and look at the sky. Now the trees covered the window, and he could not look at the sky. He fell ill—he got so sick—and the doctors could not find anything wrong with him. Because he was a man of such regularity, he was really tremendously healthy. They could not find anything wrong; they couldn't diagnose him. Then the servant said, "Don't bother, I know the reason. Those trees are intruding on his regularity. Now he cannot go to the window and sit there and look at the sky. Looking at the sky is no longer possible." The neighbor had to be persuaded. The trees were cut, and then Kant was OK; the illness disappeared.

But this is obsession. No need to become obsessive; everything has to be done with understanding.

Niyam and *asan,* regularity and posture—they are for the body. A controlled body is a beautiful phenomenon. A controlled energy, glowing, and always more than is needed and always alive, never dull and dead—then the body also becomes intelligent; the body also becomes wise; the body glows with a new awareness.

Then *pranayam* is a bridge. Deep breathing is the bridge from mind to body. You can change the body through breathing and you can change the mind through breathing. *Pratyahar* and *dharana,* returning home and concentration—belong to the transformation of the mind. Then *dhyan* is again a bridge from mind to the self—or to the "no-self," whatever you choose to call it; it is both. *Dhyan* is the bridge to *samadhi.*

The society is there—from the society to you there is a bridge, *yam.* The body is there—for the body, regularity and posture. Again there is a bridge because of the different dimension of mind from the body: *pranayam.* Then the training of the mind—*pratyahar* and *dharna,* returning back home and concentration. Then again a bridge—and this is the last bridge: *dhyan.* And then you reach the goal, *samadhi.*

Samadhi is a beautiful word. It means now everything is solved. It means *samadhan,* everything is achieved. Now there is no desire; nothing is left to achieve. There is no "beyond." You have come home.

5

POSTURE AND BREATH

Posture should be steady and comfortable.
Posture is mastered by relaxation of effort and meditation on the unlimited.
When posture is mastered, there is a cessation of the disturbances caused by dualities.
The next step after the perfection of posture is breath control, which is accomplished through holding the breath on inhalation and exhalation or stopping the breath suddenly.
The duration and frequency of the controlled breaths are conditioned by time and place, and they become more prolonged and subtle.
There is a fourth sphere of breath control, which is internal, and it goes beyond the other three.

JUST the other day, I was reading an old Indian fable, the fable of the woodcutter. The story goes this way:

> An old woodcutter was coming back from the forest carrying a big, heavy load of wood on his head. He was very old, very tired—not only tired of the day's routine work but also tired of life itself. Life had not meant much to him, just a weary round that was the same every day. Going to the forest early in the morning, the whole day cutting the wood, then carrying the load back to town by the evening. He could not remember anything else, only

this. And only this had been the whole of his life. He was bored. Life had not been a meaningful thing to him; it carried no significance.

Particularly on that day, he was very tired, perspiring. It was hard to breathe, carrying the load and himself. Suddenly, as a symbolic act, he threw down the load of wood. That moment comes to everybody's life, when one wants to throw down the load. Not only that bundle of wood on his head, it had become a symbolic act: He threw with it the whole of his life. He fell to the ground on his knees, looked at the sky, and said, "Ah, Death! You come to everybody, but why don't you come to me? What more suffering have I to see? What more burdens have I still to carry? Am I not punished enough? And what wrong have I committed?"

He could not believe his eyes—suddenly Death appeared! The woodcutter looked around, very much shocked. Whatever he had said, he never meant it! And he had never heard of anything like this—that you call Death, and Death comes.

And Death said, "Did you call me?"

The old man suddenly forgot all weariness, all tiredness, the whole life of dead routine. He jumped up, and he said, "Yes . . . yes, I called you. Please, could you help me to put the load of wood, the burden, back on my head? Seeing nobody else here, I called you."

There are moments when you are tired of life. There are moments when you would like to die. But dying is an art; it has to be learned. And to be weary of life does not really mean that deep down the lust for life has disappeared. You may be weary of a particular life, but you are not weary of life *as such*. Everybody becomes tired of a particular life—the dead routine, the weary round, the same thing again and again, a repetition. But you are not weary of life itself. And if Death comes, you will do the same as the woodcutter did. He behaved perfectly humanly; don't laugh at him. Many times you have also thought to be finished with all this nonsense that goes on. Why continue it? But if Death suddenly appears, you will not be ready.

Only a yogi can be ready to die because only a yogi knows that through a voluntary death, a willing death, the infinite life is attained. Only a yogi knows that death is a door; it is not the end. In fact, it is the beginning. In fact, beyond it open the infinities of godliness. In fact, beyond it you are for the first time really, authentically alive. Not only the physical part of your heart throbs, *you* throb. Not only are you excited by outer things, you are made ecstatic by the inner being. Life abundant, life eternal, is entered through the door of death.

Only a yogi knows that death is a door; it is not the end. In fact, it is the beginning. In fact, beyond it open the infinities of godliness.

Everybody dies—but then death is not voluntary; then death is forced on you. You are unwilling: You resist, you cry, you weep; you would like to linger a little longer on this earth in this body. You are afraid. You can't see anything except darkness, except the end. Everybody dies unwillingly, but then death is not a door. Then you close your eyes in fear.

For the people who are on the path of yoga, death is a willing phenomenon; they will it. They are not suicidal. They are not against life, they are for greater life. They sacrifice their life for a greater life. They sacrifice their ego for a greater self. They sacrifice their self, also, for the supreme self. They go on sacrificing the limited for the unlimited. And this is what growth is all about: to go on sacrificing that which you have for that which becomes possible only when you are empty, when you don't have anything.

Patanjali's whole art is of how to attain the state where you can die willingly, surrender willingly, with no resistance. These sutras are a preparation, a preparation to die and a preparation to enter a greater life.

Posture should be steady and comfortable.

Patanjali's yoga has been very much misunderstood and misinterpreted. Patanjali is not a gymnast, but yoga looks like it is gymnastics of the body. Patanjali is not against the body. He is not a man to teach you contortions of the body. He teaches you the grace of the body because he knows that only in a graceful body a graceful mind exists; only in a graceful mind a graceful self becomes possible; and only in a graceful self, the beyond.

Step by step, a deeper and higher grace has to be attained. Grace of the body is what Patanjali calls *asan,* posture. He's not a masochist. He is not teaching you to torture your body—he is not a bit against the body. How can he be? He knows the body is going to be the very foundation stone. He knows that if you miss the body, if you don't train the body, then higher training will not be possible.

The body is just like a musical instrument. It has to be rightly tuned; only then will the higher music arise out of it. If the very instrument is somehow not in a right shape and order, then how can you imagine or hope that the great harmony will arise out of it? Only discordance will arise. Body is a *veena,* a musical instrument.

The posture should be steady and should be very, very blissful, comfortable. So never try to distort your body, and never try to achieve postures that are uncomfortable.

For Westerners, sitting on the ground, sitting in *padmasan,* the lotus posture, is difficult. Their bodies have not been trained for it. There is no need to bother about it! Patanjali will not force that posture on you. In the East, from their very birth people are sitting in this way; small children are sitting on the ground. In the West, in all the cold countries, chairs are needed; the ground is too cold. But there is no need to be worried about it. If you look at Patanjali's definition of what a posture is, you will understand: It should be steady and comfortable.

If you can be steady and comfortable in a chair, it is perfectly OK—no need to try a lotus posture and force your body unnecessarily. In fact, if a Western person tries to attain to the lotus posture, it takes six months to force the body—and it is a torture. There is no need. Patanjali is not in any way trying to help or persuade you to torture the body. You *can* sit in a tortured posture, but then it will not be a posture according to Patanjali.

A posture should be such that you can forget your body. What is comfort? When you forget your body, you are comfortable. When you are reminded continuously of the body, you are uncomfortable. So whether you sit in a chair or you sit on the ground, that's not the point. Be comfortable because if you are not comfortable in the body, you cannot long for other blessings that belong to deeper layers. If the first layer is missed, all other layers are closed. If you really want to

A posture should be such that you can forget your body. What is comfort? When you forget your body, you are comfortable.

be happy, blissful, then start from the very beginning to be blissful. Comfort of the body is a basic need for anybody who is trying to reach inner ecstasies.

Posture should be steady and comfortable.

And whenever a posture is comfortable, it is bound to be steady. You fidget if the posture is uncomfortable. You go on changing sides if the posture is uncomfortable. If the posture is really comfortable, what is the need to fidget and feel restless and go on changing again and again?

And remember, the posture that is comfortable to you may not be comfortable to your neighbor, so please never teach your posture to anybody. Every body is unique. Something that is comfortable to you may be uncomfortable to somebody else.

Every body has to be unique because every body is carrying a unique soul. Your thumbprints are unique; you cannot find anybody else anywhere in the world whose thumbprints are just like yours. And not only today—you cannot find anybody in the whole past history whose thumbprints would be like yours. And those who know about these things say that even in the future there will never be a person whose thumbprint will be like yours. A thumbprint is nothing, insignificant, but that, too, is unique. That shows that every body carries a unique being. If your thumbprint is so different from others, your body—the whole body—has to be different.

So never listen to anybody's advice. You have to find your own posture. There is no need to go to any teacher to learn it; your own feeling of comfort should be the teacher. And if you try—within a few days try all the postures that you know, all the ways that you can sit—one day you will fall upon, stumble upon, the right posture. And the moment you feel the right posture, everything will become silent and calm within you. And nobody else can teach you because nobody can know how your body harmony, in what posture, will exactly be steady and comfortable.

> You have to find your own posture. Three is no need to go to any teacher to learn it; your own feeling of comfort should be the teacher.

Try to find your own posture. Try to find your own yoga. And never follow a rule because rules are averages. In a given city there are one million people: Somebody is five feet tall, somebody five five, somebody five six, somebody six feet, somebody six and a half feet. One million people, including children—you add up their heights, and then you divide the total height of one million people by one million; then you will come to an average height. It may be four feet eight inches or something. Then you go and search for the average person—you will never find them. The average person never exists. "Average" is the falsest thing in the world. Nobody is average; everybody is himself. "Average" is a mathematical thing; it is not real, it is not actual.

All rules exist for the average. They are good for understanding a certain thing, but never follow these rules; otherwise you will feel uncomfortable. Four feet eight inches is the average height—now, *you* are five feet tall, four inches taller. Cut it down. Uncomfortable! Walk in such a way that you look like the average: You will become an ugly phenomenon, a cripple; you will be like a camel, crooked everywhere. One who tries to follow the average will miss.

Average is a mathematical phenomenon, and mathematics does not exist in reality. It exists only in man's mind. If you try to find mathematics in reality you will not find it. That's why mathematics is the only perfect science—because it is absolutely unreal.

Only with unreality can you be perfect. Reality does not bother about your rules and regulations; reality moves on its own. Mathematics is a perfect science because it is mental, it is human. If man disappears from the earth, mathematics will be the first thing to disappear. Other things may continue, but mathematics cannot be here.

> Reality does not bother about your rules and regulations; reality moves on its own. Mathematics is a perfect science because it is mental, it is human.

Always remember: All rules, all disciplines, are based on the average—and the average is nonexistential. Don't try to become the average—nobody can. One has to find one's own way. Learn the average—that will be helpful—but don't make it a rule. Let it be just a tacit understanding. Just understand it, and forget about it. It will be helpful as a vague guide, not as an absolutely certain teacher. It will be just like a vague map, not perfect. That vague map will give you certain hints, but you have to find your own inner comfort, steadiness. How you feel should be the determining factor. That's why Patanjali gives this definition, so that you can discover your own feeling. There cannot be any better definition of posture:

Posture should be steady and comfortable.

In fact, I would like to say it the other way, and the Sanskrit definition can be translated in the other way: Posture is that which is steady and comfortable. *Sthir sukham asanam:* That which is steady and comfortable is posture. And that will be a more accurate translation. The moment you bring in "should," things become difficult. In the Sanskrit definition there is no "should," but in English it enters.

I have looked into many translations of Patanjali. They always say, "Posture should be steady and comfortable." In the Sanskrit definition—*sthir sukham asanam*—there is no "should." *Sthir* means "steady," *sukham* means "comfortable," *asanam* means "posture"—that's all. "Steady, comfortable: That is the posture."

Why does this "should" come in? Because we would like to make a rule out of it. It is a simple definition, an indicator, a pointer—it is not a rule. And remember it always: People like Patanjali never give rules; they are not so foolish. They simply give pointers, hints. You have to decode the hint into your own being. You have to feel it, work it out; then you will come to the rule. But that rule will be only for you, nobody else.

People like Patanjali give pointers, hints. You have to decode the hint into your own being. You have to feel it, work it out; then you will come to the rule. But that rule will be only for you, nobody else.

If people can remember this, the world will be a very beautiful world—nobody trying to force anybody to do something, nobody trying to discipline anybody else. Because your discipline may have proved good for you, but it may be poisonous for somebody else. Your medicine is not necessarily a medicine for all. Don't go on giving it to others.

But foolish people always live by rules.

I have heard that Mulla Nasruddin was learning medicine with a great physician, and he watched his master to find hints. When the master would go on his rounds to see patients, Mulla would follow. One day Mulla was surprised: The master took the pulse of a patient, closed his eyes, meditated, and said, "You have been eating too many mangoes."

Mulla was surprised. How could the master find this out through the pulse? He had never heard that anybody could find out through the pulse that somebody had been eating mangoes. He was puzzled. On the way back home he asked, "Master, please give me a little hint. How could you . . . ?"

The master laughed; he said, "The pulse cannot show this, but I looked under the bed of the patient. There were many mangoes, some uneaten and a few scraps. So I just inferred; it was an inference."

The master was ill one day, so Mulla had to go in his place for the daily rounds. He went to see a new patient, took the pulse in his hand, closed his eyes, brooded a little—just exactly like the master—and then he said, "You have been eating too many horses."

The patient said, "What!? Are you mad?"

Mulla was very puzzled. He came home very disturbed and sad. The master asked, "What happened?"

Mulla said, "I, too, looked under the bed. A saddle and other things were there—the horse was not there—so I thought, 'He has eaten too many horses.' "

This is how the stupid mind goes on following. Don't be stupid. Take these definitions, sayings, sutras, in a very vague way. Let them become part of your understanding, but don't try to follow them exactly. Let them go deep in you, so they become your intelligence, and then seek *your* path. All great teaching is indirect.

How to attain to this posture? How to attain this steadiness? First look at the comfort. If your body is exactly in deep comfort, in deep rest, feeling good, a certain well-being surrounds you—that should be the criterion with which to judge. That should become the touchstone. And this is possible while you are standing; this is possible while you are lying down; this is possible while you are sitting on the ground or sitting on a chair. It is possible anywhere because it is an inner feeling of comfort. And whenever it is attained, you will not want to continue moving again and again because the more you move, the more you will miss it. It happens in a certain state. If you move, you move away from it; you disturb it.

The natural desire in everybody—and yoga is the most natural thing—is to be comfortable. Whenever you are in discomfort you will want to change it—that is natural. Always listen to the natural, instinctive mechanism within you. It is almost always correct.

Posture is mastered by relaxation of effort and meditation on the unlimited.

Beautiful words, great indicators, and pointers. *Prayantna shaithilya*—relaxation of effort—is the first thing if you want to attain what Patanjali calls a posture. Comfortable, steady, the body in such deep stillness that nothing moves. The body so comfortable that the desire to move disappears; you start enjoying the feeling of comfort, and it becomes steady.

And with the change of your mood, the body changes; with the change of the body, your mood changes. Have you ever watched it? You go to a theater, a movie: Have you watched how many times you change your posture? Have you tried to correlate it? If there is something very sensational happening on the screen, you cannot sit leaning back against the chair. You sit up, your spine becomes straight. If something boring is going on and you are not excited, you relax. Now your spine is no longer straight. If something very uncomfortable is going on, you go on changing your posture. If something is really beautiful there, even your eye blinking stops; even that much movement will be a disturbance—no movement, you become completely steady, restful, as if the body has disappeared.

The first thing to attain to this posture is the relaxation of effort, which is one of the most difficult things in the world—the most simple, yet most difficult. Simple to attain if you understand; very difficult to attain if you don't understand. It is not a question of practice, it is a question of understanding.

In the West, Emile Coué has discovered a particular law that he calls the law of reverse effect. It is one of the most fundamental things in the human mind. There are things that you may want to do, but please don't try to do them; otherwise the reverse will be the effect.

For example, you are not falling asleep—don't *try.* If you try, sleep will be further and further away. If you try too much, it will be impossible to sleep because every effort goes against sleep. Sleep comes only when there is no effort. When you are not bothered about sleep, you are just lying down on your pillow, just enjoying the coolness of the pillow or the warmth of the blanket, the dark, velvety surrounding encompassing you, you are just enjoying it . . . nothing else. You are not even thinking about sleep. Some dreams pass through the mind: You look at them in a very, very sleepy way, not interested too much even in them because if interest arises, sleep disappears. You just somehow remain aloof, just enjoying, resting, not seeking any end—and sleep comes.

If you start trying so that sleep should come, once the "should" enters, it is almost impossible. Then you can remain awake the whole night, and if you fall asleep that may be only because you get tired of the effort. When effort is no longer there—because you have done everything, and you have given up—sleep comes in.

Emile Coué discovered the law of reverse effect only a few decades ago. Patanjali must have known it almost five thousand years ago. He talks about *prayatna shaithilya,* relaxation of the effort. You would have assumed just the reverse, that much effort should be made to attain to the right posture. Patanjali says, "If you make too much effort, it will not be possible. No-effort allows it to happen."

Effort should be relaxed completely because effort is part of the will, and will is against surrender. If you try to do something, you are not allowing existence to do it. When you give up, when you say, "OK, let thy will be done. If you are sending sleep, perfectly good. If you are not sending sleep, that, too, is perfectly good. I have no complaints to make; I am not grumbling about it. You know better. If it is needed to send sleep for me, send it. If it is not needed, perfectly good—don't send it. Please, don't listen to me! Your will should be done." This is how one relaxes effort.

Effortlessness is a great phenomenon. Once you know it, many millions of things become possible to you. Through effort, the marketplace; through effortlessness, the beyond. Through effort you can never reach nirvana—you can reach New Delhi but not nirvana.

Through effort you can attain things of the world; they are

never attained without effort, remember. So if you want to attain more riches, don't listen to me—because then you will be very, very angry with me, that this man disturbed your whole life. "He was saying, 'Stop making efforts, and many things will become possible,' and I have been sitting and waiting, and the money is not coming. Nobody is coming with an invitation to 'Come, and please become the president of the country.' "

Nobody is going to come. These foolish things are attained by effort.

If you want to become a president, you have to make a mad effort for it. Unless you go completely mad, you will never become a president of a country. You have to be madder than other competitors, remember, because you are not alone there. Great competition exists; many others also are trying. In fact, everybody else is trying to reach the same place. Much effort is needed, and don't try in a gentlemanly way; otherwise you will be defeated. No gentlemanliness is needed there. Be rude, violent, aggressive; don't bother about what you are doing to others. Stick to your program. Even if others are killed for your power politics, let them be killed. Make everybody a ladder, a step. Go on walking on people's heads; only then do you become a president or a prime minister. There is no other way.

The ways of the world are the ways of violence and will. If you relax the will, you will be thrown out; somebody will jump on you. You will be made a means. If you want to succeed in the ways of the world, never listen to people like Patanjali; then it is better to read Machiavelli, Chanakya—cunning, the most cunning people of the world. They give you advice for how to exploit everybody and not allow anybody to exploit you, how to be ruthless, without any compassion, just violent.

Only then can you reach power, prestige, money, things of the world. But if you want to attain to things of the beyond, just the opposite is needed: no-effort. Effortlessness is needed, relaxation is needed.

It has happened many times. I have many friends in the world of politics, in the world of money, the market. They come to me and they say, "Teach us somehow to relax. We cannot relax." A minister used to come to me, and he always came with the same problem: "I cannot relax. Help me."

I told him, "If you really want to relax, you will have to leave politics. This ministership cannot go together with relaxation. If you relax, you lose. So you decide. I can teach you relaxation, but don't be angry then because these two things cannot be possible together. First be finished with your politics; then come to me."

He said, "That is not possible. I have come to learn relaxation so that I can work hard and become a chief minister. Because of these tensions in the mind and continuous worries, I cannot work hard. And others—they go on working. They are great competitors, and I am losing the battle. I have not come to you in order to leave politics."

So I said, "Then, please, don't come. Forget about me. Just be in politics, get really tired, bored, be finished with it; then come to me."

Relaxation is a totally different dimension, just the contrary.

You move in the world with will. Nietzsche has written a book, *The Will to Power*. That is the right scripture to read, *The Will to Power.* Patanjali is not about "will to power"; it is about surrender to the whole.

The first thing is *prayatna shaithilya*—effortlessness. You should simply feel comfortable. Don't make much effort around it. Let the feeling do the work; don't bring the will in. How can you force comfort on yourself? It is impossible. You can be comfortable if you allow comfort to happen. You cannot force it.

How can you force love? If you don't love a person, you don't love a person; what can you do? You can try, pretend, force yourself, but just the reverse will be the result. If you *try* to love a person, you will hate him more. The only result will be that after your efforts you will hate the person, and you will take revenge. You will say, "What type of ugly person is he? Because I am trying so much to love and nothing happens." You will make him responsible. You will make him feel guilty, as if he is doing something. He is not doing anything.

Love cannot be willed; prayer cannot be willed; posture cannot be willed. You have to feel. Feeling is a totally different thing than willing.

Buddha became a Buddha not by will. He tried for six years continually through will. He was a man of the world, trained as a prince, trained to become a king. He must have been taught everything that Chanakya had said.

Chanakya is the Indian Machiavelli—and even a little more cunning than Machiavelli because Indians have a quality of mind to go to the very roots. If they become Buddha, they *really* become Buddha. If they become Chanakya, you cannot compete with them. Wherever they go, they go to the very root. Even Machiavelli is a little immature before Chanakya. Chanakya is absolute.

Buddha must have been taught—every prince has to be taught. The name of Machiavelli's greatest book is *The Prince*. He must have been taught all the ways of the world; he was supposed to tackle with people in the world; he had to cling to his power. And then he left!

But it is easy to leave the palace; it is easy to leave the kingdom. It is difficult to leave the training of the mind. For six years he tried, through the will, to attain enlightenment. He did whatsoever is humanly possible and even inhumanly possible. He did everything; he left nothing undone.

Nothing happened.

The more he tried, the more he felt himself far away. In fact, the more he exercised the will and made efforts through it, the more he felt that he was deserted: "Enlightenment, transcendence, is nowhere." Nothing was happening.

Then one evening he gave up. That very night he became enlightened. That very night *prayatna shaithilya,* relaxation of the effort, happened. He became a Buddha not by willpower; he became a Buddha when he surrendered, when he gave up.

I teach you meditations, and I go on telling you, "Make every effort that you can make." But always remember, this emphasis on making all the efforts is just so that your will is torn apart, so that your will is finished and the dream of the will is finished. So that you are so fed up with the will that one day you simply give up. That very day you become enlightened.

But don't be in a hurry because you can give up right now without making the effort—but it will not help. That will be a cunning thing, and you cannot win with existence by being cunning. You have to be very innocent. The thing has to just happen.

These are simply definitions. Patanjali is not saying, "Do this!" He is simply defining the path. If you understand it, it will start affecting you, your way of life, your being. Absorb it, let it be saturated deep within you. Let it flow with your blood, let it become your very marrow. That's all. Forget Patanjali. These sutras are not to be crammed into your head. They should not be made part of your memory, they should become part of you.

Your total being should have the understanding, that's all. Then forget about them. They start functioning.

Posture is mastered by relaxation of effort and meditation on the unlimited.

Two points. Relax effort; don't force it, allow it to happen. It is like sleep—allow it to happen. It is a deep let-go—allow it to happen. Don't try to force it; otherwise you will kill it. And the second thing is that while the body is allowing itself to be comfortable, to settle in a deep rest, your mind should be focused on the unlimited.

The mind is very clever with the limited. If you think about money, the mind is clever; if you think about power and politics, the mind is clever; if you think about words, philosophies, systems, beliefs, the mind is clever—these are all limited. If you think about God, there is suddenly a vacuum. . . . What can you think about God? If you can think, then that God is no longer God; it has become limited. If you can think of God as Krishna, it is no longer God. Krishna may then be standing there singing on his flute, but there is a limitation. If you think of God as Christ—finished! God is no longer there; you have made a limited being out of it. Beautiful—but nothing to be compared with the beauty of the unlimited.

There are two types of God. One is the God of belief—the Christian God, Hindu God, Mohammedan God. The other is the God of reality, not of belief—that is unlimited, that is godliness itself. If you think about the Mohammedan God, you will be a Mohammedan but not a religious man. If you think about the Christian God, you will be a Christian but not a religious man. If you just bring your mind to godliness, you will be religious—no longer Hindu, no longer Mohammedan, no longer Christian.

There are two types of God. One is the God of belief—the Christian God, Hindu God, Mohammedan God. The other is the God of reality, not of belief—that is unlimited, that is godliness itself.

And that godliness is not a concept! A concept is a toy your mind can play with. The real God is so vast—it is godliness that plays with your mind, not your mind playing with God. Then God is no longer a toy in your hands; you are a toy in the hands of the godliness. The whole thing has totally changed. Now you are no longer controlling the situation, you are no longer in control. Godliness has taken possession of you.

The right term is "to be possessed"—to be possessed by the infinite. It is no longer a picture before your mind's eye. No, there is no picture. Vast emptiness . . . and in that vast emptiness you are dissolving. Not only is any definition of God lost, all boundaries are lost; when you come in contact with the infinite, you start losing your boundaries. Your boundaries become vague, your boundaries become less and less certain, more flexible; you are disappearing like smoke into the sky. A moment comes when you look at yourself . . . and you are not there.

So Patanjali says two things: No effort, and consciousness focused on the infinite. That's how you attain to *asan*. And this is only the beginning; this is only the body. One has to go deeper.

When posture is mastered, there is a cessation of the disturbances caused by dualities.

When the body is really in comfort, restful . . . the flame of the body is not wavering; it has become steady, there is no movement . . . suddenly, as if time has stopped, no winds blowing, everything still and calm, and the body has no urge to move. Settled, deeply balanced, tranquil, quiet, collected—in that state, dualities and the disturbances caused by dualities disappear.

Have you observed that whenever your mind is disturbed, your body fidgets more? You cannot sit silently. Or whenever your body is fidgeting, your mind cannot be silent. They are together.

Have you observed that whenever your mind is disturbed, your body fidgets more? You cannot sit silently. Or whenever your body is fidgeting, your mind cannot be silent. They are together. Patanjali knows well that body and mind are not two things; you are not divided in two, body and mind. Body and mind are one thing. You are psychosomatic, you are "bodymind." The body is just the beginning of your mind, and the mind is nothing but the end of the body. Both are two aspects of one phenomenon; they are not two.

So whatever happens in the body affects the mind, and whatever happens in the mind affects the body. They run parallel. That's why so much emphasis is on the body—because if your body is not in deep rest, your mind cannot be.

And it is easier to start with the body because that is the outermost layer. It is difficult to start with the mind. Many people try to start with the mind and fail because their body will not cooperate. It is always best to begin from ABC and go slowly, in the right sequence. Body is first, the beginning; one should start with the body. If you can attain tranquility of the body, suddenly you will see the mind is falling in order.

Mind moves to the left and to the right, like a pendulum of an old grandfather clock, continuously, right to left . . . left to right. And if you observe a pendulum, you will know something about your mind. When the pendulum is moving toward the left, visibly it is going to the left, but invisibly it is gaining momentum to go to the right. When the eyes say that the pendulum is going to the left, that very movement toward the left creates the momentum, the energy, for the pendulum to go to the right, again. When it is going to the right, it is again building energy, gaining energy to go to the left.

So whenever you are in love, you are gaining energy to hate. Whenever you are in hate, you are gaining energy to love. Whenever you are feeling happy, you are gaining energy to feel unhappy. Whenever you are feeling unhappy, you are gaining energy to feel happy. This is how the momentum continues.

This is the situation of your mind, continually moving from one extreme to another—leftist, rightist, leftist, rightist, never in the middle. And to be in the middle is really to be. Both extremes are burdensome because you cannot be comfortable. In the middle is comfort because in the middle the weight disappears. Exactly in the middle, you become weightless. Move to the left, and the weight enters; move to the right and the weight enters. And go on moving. . . . The farther away you move from the middle, the more weight you will have to carry.

Be in the middle. A religious person is neither leftist nor

rightist. A religious person does not follow the extremes; he is a man of no extreme. And when you are exactly in the middle—your body and your mind both—all dualities disappear. All dualities exist because *you* are dual, because you go on leaning from this side to that.

When posture is mastered, there is a cessation of the disturbances caused by dualties.

And when there is no duality, how can you be tense? How can you be in agony, how can you be in conflict? When there are two within you, there is conflict. They go on fighting, and they will never leave you at rest. Your home is divided; you are always in a civil war. You live in a fever. When this duality disappears, you become silent, centered, in the middle. Buddha has called his way *Majjhim Nikaya,* the middle way. He used to tell his disciples, "The only thing to be followed is this: Always be in the middle; don't go to the extremes."

There are extremists all over the world. Somebody is chasing women all the time—a Romeo, a Casanova, continuously chasing women. And then someday he becomes frustrated with all the chasing. Then he leaves the world; then he becomes a *sannyasin.* And then he teaches everybody to be against women and goes on saying, "A woman is hell. Be alert! A woman is only a trap." Whenever you find a *sannyasin* talking against women, you can know he must have been a Romeo before. He is not saying anything about women; he is saying something about his past. Now one extreme is finished; he has moved to another extreme.

Somebody is mad after money. And many are mad, just obsessed, as if their whole life is to make bigger and bigger piles of dollars. It seems to be their only reason to be here, that when they go to death they will leave big piles—bigger than those of others. That seems to be their whole significance. When such a man becomes frustrated, he will go on teaching, "Money is the enemy." Whenever you find somebody teaching that money is the enemy, you can know that this man must have been money mad. He is still mad—at the opposite extreme.

A really balanced man is not against anything because he is not *for* anything. If you come and ask me, "Are you against money?" I can only shrug my shoulders. I am not against it because I have never been for it. Money is a utility, a medium of exchange—no need to be mad about it either way. Use it if you have it. If you don't have it, enjoy the nonhaving of it. If you have it, use it. If you don't have it then enjoy that state. That's all a man of understanding will do. If he lives in a palace, he enjoys; if there is no palace, then he enjoys the hut. Whatsoever is the case, he is happy and balanced. He is neither for the palace nor against it.

A man who is for *and* against is lopsided; he is not balanced.

Buddha used to say to his disciples, "Just be balanced, and everything else will become possible of its own accord. Just be in the middle." And that is what Patanjali says when he is talking about the posture. The outer posture is of the body, the inner posture is of the mind; they are connected. When the body is in the middle—restful, steady—the mind is also in the middle, restful, steady. When the body is in rest, body feeling disappears; when the mind is in rest, mind feeling disappears. Then you are only the soul, the transcendental, which is neither the body nor the mind.

The next step after the perfection of posture is breath control, which is accomplished through holding the breath on inhalation and exhalation, or stopping the breath suddenly.

Between body and mind, breath is the bridge—these three things have to be understood. Body posture, mind merging into the infinite, and the bridge that joins them together—all have to be in a right rhythm. Have you observed? If not, then observe that whenever your mind changes, the breathing changes. The reverse is also true: Change your breathing, and the mind changes.

When you are deep in sexual passion, have you noticed how you breathe? Very nonrhythmic, feverish, excited. If you continue breathing that way, you will soon be tired, exhausted. It will not give you life; in fact, in that way you are losing some life. When you are calm and quiet, feeling happy, suddenly one morning or evening looking at the stars, nothing to do, a holiday, just resting—look, watch the breathing. The breathing is so peaceful you cannot even feel it, whether it is moving or not. When you are angry, watch. The breathing changes immediately. When you feel love, watch. When you are sad, watch. With every mood the breathing has a different rhythm: it is a bridge.

When you are angry, watch. The breathing changes immediately. When you feel love, watch. When you are sad, watch. With every mood the breathing has a different rhythm.

When your body is healthy, breathing has a different quality. When your body is ill, the breathing is ill. When you are in perfect health, you completely forget about breathing. When you are not in perfect health, the breathing comes again and again to your notice; something is wrong.

The next step after the perfection of posture is breath control . . .

This term "breath control" is not good; it is not a correct rendering of the word *pranayam. Pranayam* never means breath control. It simply means the expansion of the vital energy. *Prana-ayam—prana* means the vital energy hidden in breath, and *ayam* means infinite expansion. It is not "breath control." The very word *control* is a little ugly because it gives you a feeling of the *controller*—the will enters. *Pranayam* is totally different—expansion of vitality, breathing in such a way that you become one with the breathing of the whole. Breathing in such a way that you are not breathing in your own individual way, you are breathing with the whole.

Try this; sometimes it happens: Two lovers sitting by each other's side, holding hands—if they are really in love, they will suddenly become aware that they are breathing simultaneously, they are breathing together. They are not breathing separately. When the woman inhales, the man inhales. When the man exhales, the woman exhales. Try it. Sometime, suddenly become aware: If you are sitting with a friend, you will be breathing together. If the enemy is sitting there, and you want to get rid of him, or some bore is there, and you want to get rid of him, you will be breathing separately; you will never breathe in rhythm.

Sit with a tree. If you are silent, enjoying, delighting, suddenly you will become aware that the tree, somehow, is breathing the same way you are breathing.

And there comes a moment when one feels that one is breathing together with the whole; one becomes the breath of the whole. One is no longer fighting, struggling; one is surrendered. One is with the whole—so much so, that there is no need to breathe separately.

In deep love, people breathe together—in hatred, never. I have a feeling that if you are inimical to somebody, he may be a thousand miles away. This is just a feeling because no scientific research exists for it, but someday such scientific research is possible. I have a very deep feeling that if you are inimical to somebody—he may be in America, and you may be in India—you will breathe separately, you cannot breathe together. And your lover may be in China, you may be on another continent—you may not even have the address of where your lover is—but you will breathe together. This is how it should be, and I know it is that way, but no scientific proof exists. That's why I say this is just my feeling. Someday someday will also prove the scientific aspect.

There are a few proofs that suggest this. For example, in Russia there have been a few experiments with telepathy. Two persons—separate, far away, hundreds of miles away—one person is the broadcaster, and the other is the receiver in the experiment. At a fixed time, twelve in the afternoon, one starts sending messages. He makes a copy of a triangle, concentrates on it, and sends the message: "I have made a triangle." And the other person tries to receive, just remains open, feeling, groping: What message is coming? And the scientists have observed that if he receives the triangle, then the two people are breathing in the same way; if he misses the triangle, then they are not breathing in the same way.

In deep breathing together, something of deep empathy arises; you become one—because breath is life. Then feeling can be transferred, thoughts can be transferred.

If you go to meet a saint, always watch his breathing. And if you feel sympathetic, in deep love with him, watch your breathing also. You will suddenly feel that the nearer you come to him, your feeling and your breathing fall in tune with his breathing.

Aware or unaware, that is not the point; but it happens. When you are in sympathy you breathe together. It simply happens by itself; some unknown law functions.

Pranayam means to breathe with the whole. That is my translation, not "control of breath" but to breathe with the whole. It is absolutely uncontrolled! If you control, how can you breathe with the whole? So to translate *pranayam* as "breath control" is a misunderstanding. It is not only incorrect, inadequate, it is certainly wrong. Just the opposite is the case.

To breathe with the whole, to become the breath of the eternal and the whole, is *pranayam*. Then you expand.

To breathe with the whole, to become the breath of the eternal and the whole, is *pranayam*. Then you expand. Then your life energy goes on expanding with the trees and mountains and sky and stars. Then a moment comes, the day you become a buddha . . . you have completely disappeared. Now you no longer breathe; the whole breathes in you. Now your breathing and the whole's breathing are never apart; they are always together. So much so that it is now useless to say, "This is my breath."

The next step after the perfection of posture is breath control—*pranayam*—which is accomplished through holding the breath on inhalation and exhalation or stopping the breath suddenly.

When you breathe in, there comes a moment when the breath has completely gone in—for a certain second the breathing stops. The same happens when you exhale. When you breathe out—when the breath is completely released—for a certain second again the breathing stops. In those moments you face death, and to face death is to face the eternal. I repeat: To face death is to face the eternal because when you die, the eternal lives in you. Only after crucifixion is there resurrection. That's why I say Patanjali is teaching the art of dying.

When the breathing stops, when there is no breathing, you are in exactly the same state as you will be in when you die. For a second you are in tune with death—breathing has stopped. The whole of *The Book of Secrets, Vigyan Bhairav Tantra* is concerned with it—emphatically concerned with it—because if you can enter into that stoppage, there is the door.

It is very subtle and narrow. Jesus has said again and again, "Narrow is my way—straight but narrow, very narrow." Kabir has said, "Two cannot pass together, only one." So narrow that if you are a crowd inside, you cannot pass. If you are even divided in two—left and right—you cannot pass. If you become one, a unison, a harmony, then you can pass.

Narrow is the way. Straight, of course—it is not a crooked thing; it goes directly to the temple of the divine—but very narrow. You cannot take anybody with you. You cannot take your things with you. You cannot take your knowledge, you cannot take your sacrifices, you cannot take your woman, your man, your children. You cannot take anybody. In fact, you cannot take even your ego, even yourself. You will pass through it, but everything else other than your purest being has to be left at the door.

Yes, narrow is the way. Straight but narrow.

And these are the moments to find the way. When the breath goes in and stops for a second, when the breath goes out and stops for a second, attune yourself to become more and more aware of these stops, these gaps. Through these gaps the eternal enters you like death.

Somebody was telling me, "In the West, we don't have any parallel to *Yama,* the god of death." He was asking me, "Why do you call death a god? Death is the enemy. Why should death be called a god? If you call death the devil, it is OK, but why do you call it a god?"

I said we call it a god very deliberately—because death is the door to God. In fact, death is deeper than the life that you know. Not the life that I know, but your death is deeper than your life, and when you move through that death you will come to a life that doesn't belong to you or me or to anybody. It is the life of the whole, and death is the god.

A whole Upanishad exists, the *Kathopanishad*—the whole story, the whole parable, is that a small child is sent to Death to learn the secret of life. Absurd, patently absurd: Why go to Death to learn the secret of life? It looks like a paradox, but it is the reality. If you want to know life—real life—you will have to ask Death because when your so-called life stops, only then does real life function.

The next step after the perfection of posture is* pranayam*, which is accomplished through holding the breath.

So when you inhale, hold it a little longer so that the gate can be felt. When you exhale, hold the breath outside a little longer so that you can feel the gap a little more easily. You have a little more time.

. . . or stopping the breath suddenly.

Or, anytime, stop the breath suddenly. Walking on the road, stop it—just a sudden jerk, and death enters. Anytime, anywhere you can stop the breath suddenly—in that stopping, death enters.

The duration and frequency of the controlled breaths are conditioned by time and place and become more prolonged and subtle.

The more you do these stoppages, these gaps, the more the gate becomes a little wider, and you can feel it more. Try it, make it a part of your life. Whenever you are not doing anything, let the breath go in . . . and stop it. Feel it—somewhere there is the door. It is dark, so you will have to grope; the door is not immediately available. You will have to grope for it, but you will find it.

And whenever you stop the breath, thoughts will stop immediately. Try it. Suddenly stop the breath—and immediately there is a break and thoughts stop because thoughts and breaths both belong to life, this so-called life. In the other life, the transcendental life, breathing is not needed. You live—there is no need to breathe. And thoughts are not needed. You live—thoughts are not needed. Thoughts and breath are part of the physical world. No-thought and no-breath are part of the eternal world.

There is a fourth sphere of breath control, which is internal, and it goes beyond the other three.

Patanjali says there are these three things—stopping inside, stopping outside, stopping suddenly—and there is also a fourth, which is internal. Buddha has emphasized that fourth thing very much; he calls it *anapanasata* yoga. He says, "Don't try to stop anywhere. Simply watch the whole process of breath." The breath is coming in—you watch, don't miss a single point; the breath is coming in, you go on watching. Then there is a stop, an automatic stop when the breath has entered you—watch the stop. Don't do anything, simply be a watcher. Then the breath starts on the outer journey—go on watching. When the breath is completely out, it stops—watch that stop, too. Then the breath goes on coming in, going out, coming in, going out—you simply watch. This is the fourth: Just by watching, you become separate from the breath.

When you are separate from the breath you are separate from the thoughts. In fact, breath is the process in the body that is parallel to thoughts in the mind. Thoughts move in the mind, breath moves in the body. They are parallel forces, two aspects of the same coin. Patanjali also refers to it, although he has not emphasized the fourth. He simply refers to it, but Buddha has completely focused his whole attention on the fourth; he never talks about the other three. The whole of Buddhist meditation is the fourth.

There is a fourth sphere of* pranayam—that is of witnessing—*which is internal, and it goes beyond the other three.

But Patanjali is really very scientific. He never uses the fourth, but he says that it is beyond the three. Must be that Patanjali didn't have as beautiful a group of disciples as Buddha had. Patanjali must have been working with more body-oriented people, and Buddha was working with more mind-oriented people. Patanjali says that the fourth goes beyond the three, even though he himself never uses it. He goes on saying all that can be said about yoga. He is the alpha and the omega, the beginning and the end; he has not left out a single point. Patanjali's *Yoga Sutras* cannot be improved.

There are only two persons in the world who created a whole science by themselves. One is Aristotle in the West, who created the science of logic—alone, with nobody's help. And for these two thousand years nothing has been improved; it remains the same. It remains perfect. Another is Patanjali, who created the whole science of yoga—which is many times, a million times, greater than logic—alone. And it could not be improved. It has not been improved, and I don't see any point where it can be improved. The whole science is there—perfect, absolutely perfect.

6

YOGA IN THE FAST LANE

Responses to Questions

Please explain how it is possible that just by looking, by witnessing the recordings in the brain cells, the sources of thought process can cease to be.

THEY never cease to be, but just by witnessing, the identification is broken. Buddha lived in his body for forty years after his enlightenment. The body did not cease; for forty years he was talking, explaining, making people understand what had happened to him and how the same could happen to them. He was using the mind; the mind had not ceased. And when he came back after twelve years to his hometown, he recognized his father, he recognized his wife, he recognized his son. The mind was there, the memory was there; otherwise recognition is impossible. The mind had not really ceased.

When we say the mind ceases, we mean your identification is broken. Now you know: This is the mind, and this is "I am." The bridge is broken. Now the mind is not the master. It has become just an instrument; it has fallen into its right place, so whenever you need it, you can use it. It is just like a fan: If you want to use it, you switch it on, and the fan starts functioning. Right now you are not using the fan, so it is nonfunctioning, but it is there. It has not ceased to be. At any moment you can use it. It has not disappeared.

Just by witnessing, identification disappears—not the mind. But with identification disappearing, you are totally a new being. For the first time you have come to know your real phenomenon, your real reality. For the first time you have come to know who you are. Now the mind is just part of the mechanism around you.

It is just as if you are a pilot and flying an airplane. You use many instruments; your eyes are working over many instruments, continuously aware of this and that. But you are not the instruments. This mind, this body, and many functions of the bodymind, are just around you—the mechanism. In this mechanism you can exist in two ways. One way of existence is forgetting yourself and feeling as if you are the mechanism. This is bondage, this is misery; this is the world, the *samsar.*

Another way of functioning is this: Become alert that you are separate, that you are different—then you go on using the mechanism, but now there is a lot of difference. Now the mechanism is not you. And if something goes wrong in the mechanism, you can try to put it right, but you will not be disturbed. Even if the whole mechanism disappears, you will not be disturbed.

Buddha dying and you dying are two different phenomena. Buddha dying knows that only the mechanism is dying. It has been used, and now there is no need. A burden has been removed; he is becoming free. He will move now without form. But you dying is totally different. You are suffering, you are crying because you feel *you* are dying, not the mechanism. It is *your* death. Then it becomes an intense suffering.

Just by witnessing, the mind doesn't cease, and the brain cells will not cease. Rather, they will become more alive because there will be less conflict, more energy. They will become fresher, and you can use them more accurately. But you will not be burdened by them, and they will not force you to do something. They will not push and pull you here and there. You will be the master.

But how does it happen just by witnessing? Because it has happened—the bondage has happened—by *not* witnessing. The bondage has happened because you are not alert, so the bondage will disappear if you become alert. The bondage is only unawareness. Nothing else is needed except becoming more alert, whatsoever you do.

You are sitting here listening to me—you can listen with awareness, or you can listen without awareness. Without awareness listening will be there, too, but it will be a different thing; the quality will differ. Then your ears are listening, but your mind is functioning somewhere else. Then somehow a few words will penetrate you, but they will be mixed, and your mind will interpret them in its own way. And it will put its own ideas into them. Everything will be a muddle and a mess. You have listened, but many things will be bypassed, many things you will not hear. You will choose. Then the whole thing will be distorted.

If you are alert, the moment you become alert, thinking ceases. With alertness you cannot think. The whole energy becomes alert; there is no energy left to move into thinking. When you are alert even for a single moment, you simply listen. There is no barrier. Your words are not there to get mixed in. You need not interpret. The impact is direct.

If you can listen with alertness, then what I am saying may be meaningful or may not be meaningful, but your listening with alertness will always be significant. That very alertness will make a peak of your consciousness. The past will dissolve; the future will disappear. You will be nowhere else; you will just be here and now. And in that moment of silence when thinking is not, you will be deep in contact with your own source. And that source is bliss—and that source is divine.

So the only thing to be done is to do everything with alertness.

You said that the spiritual endeavor may take twenty to thirty years or even lives—and that even then it is early. But the Western mind seems to be result oriented, impatient, and too practical. It wants instantaneous results. Religious techniques come and go like other fads in the West. How then do you intend to introduce yoga to the Western mind?

I am not interested in the Western mind or the Eastern mind. These are just two aspects of one mind. I am interested in the mind. And this East-West dichotomy is not very meaningful, not even significant now. There are Eastern minds in the West and there are Western minds in the East. And now the whole thing has become a mess. The East is now also in a hurry. The old East has disappeared completely.

I am reminded of a Taoist anecdote:

> Three Taoists were meditating in a cave. One year passed. They remained silent, sitting, meditating. One day a horseman passed nearby. They looked. One of the three hermits said, "The horse he was riding was white." The other two remained silent. After one year again, the second hermit said, "The horse was black, not white." Then one more year passed again. The third hermit said, "If there is going to be any bickering, I am leaving. I am leaving! You are disturbing my silence!"

What did it matter whether the horse was white or black? Three years! But this was the flow in the East. Time was not. The

East was not conscious of time at all. The East lived in eternity, as if time were not passing. Everything was static.

But that East no longer exists. The West has corrupted everything, and the East has disappeared. Through Western education everybody is now Western. Only a few islandlike people are left who are Eastern—they can be in the West, they can be in the East; they are not in any way confined to the East. But the world as a whole, the earth as a whole, has become Western.

Yoga says—and let it penetrate you very deeply because it will be very meaningful—yoga says that the more you are impatient, the more time will be needed for your transformation. The more you are in a hurry, the more you will be delayed. Hurry itself creates such a confusion that delay will result.

Yoga says that the more you are impatient, the more time will be needed for your transformation. The more you are in a hurry, the more you will be delayed.

The less you are in a hurry, the earlier will be the results. If you are infinitely patient, this very moment transformation can happen. If you are ready to wait forever, you may not have to wait even for the next moment. This very moment the thing can happen because it is not a question of time; it is a question of your quality of the mind.

Infinite patience . . . Simply not hankering for results gives you much depth. Hurry makes you shallow. You are in such a hurry that you cannot be deep. This moment you are not interested here, in this moment, but rather what is going to happen in the next. You are interested in results. You are moving ahead of yourself; your movement is mad. So you may run too much, you may travel too much—you will not reach anywhere because the goal to be reached is just here. You have to drop into it, not to reach anywhere. And the dropping in is possible only if you are totally patient.

I will tell you one Zen anecdote:

A Zen monk is passing through a forest. Suddenly he becomes aware that a tiger is following him, so he starts running. But his running is also of a Zen type; he is not in a hurry. He is not mad. His running is smooth, harmonious. He is enjoying it. And the monk thinks in the mind, "If the tiger is enjoying it, then why not I?"

Then he comes near a precipice. Just to escape from the tiger, he hangs on to the branch of a tree. And then he looks downward. A lion is standing there in the valley, waiting for him. Then the tiger has come; he is standing just near the tree on the hilltop. And the monk is hanging in between, just from a branch, and a lion is waiting for him, deep down below.

He laughs. Then he looks more closely. Two mice are gnawing through the branch—one white, one black. The monk laughs very loudly. He says, "This is life. Day and night, white and black mice. And wherever I go, death is waiting. This is life!" And it is said that he achieves a *satori,* the first glimpse of enlightenment. This is life! Nothing to worry about; this is how things go. Wherever you go, death is waiting—and even if you don't go anywhere, day and night are cutting your life. So he laughs.

Then he looks around because now it is fixed. Now there is no worry. When death is certain, what is the worry? Only in uncertainty is there worry. When every-

> thing is certain, there is no worry; now it has become a destiny. So he looks for how to enjoy these few moments. He becomes aware that just by the side of the branch are some strawberries, so he picks a few strawberries, eats them. They are the best of his life. He enjoys them, and it is said he becomes enlightened in that moment.
>
> He has become a buddha because death is so near—and even then he is not in any hurry. He can enjoy a strawberry. It is sweet! The taste of it is sweet! He thanks existence. It is said that in that moment, everything disappears—the tiger, the lion, the branch, and he himself. He has become the cosmos.

This is patience, absolute patience! Wherever you are, in that moment enjoy it without asking for the future. No futuring in the mind—just the present moment, the nowness of the moment, and you are satisfied. Then there is no need to go anywhere. Wherever you are, from that very point you will drop into the ocean; you will become one with the cosmos.

But the mind is not interested in here and now. The mind is interested somewhere in the future, in some results. So the question is, in a way, relevant for such a mind—the modern mind it will be better to call it, rather than Western. The modern mind is constantly obsessed with the future, with the result, not with the here and now.

How can this mind be taught yoga? This mind can be taught yoga because this future orientation is leading nowhere. And this future orientation is creating constant misery for the modern mind. We have created a hell, and we have created too much of it. Now either man will have to disappear from this planet Earth, or he will have to transform himself. Either humanity will have to die completely—because this hell cannot be continued anymore—or we will have to go through a mutation.

Hence, yoga can become very meaningful and significant for the modern mind because yoga can save you. It can teach you again how to be here and now—how to forget past, how to forget future, and how to remain in the present moment with such intensity that this moment becomes timeless; the very moment becomes eternity.

Patanjali can become more and more significant. In the coming years, techniques for human transformation will become more and more important. They are already becoming so all over the world—whether you call them yoga or Zen, or you call them Sufi methods or Tantra methods, in many, many ways, all the old traditional teachings are erupting. Some deep need is there, and those who are thinking—anywhere, in any part of the world—have become interested to find again how humanity in the past existed with such beatitude, such bliss. With such poor conditions, how did such rich men exist in the past while we, with such a rich situation, why are we so poor?

This is a paradox, the modern paradox. For the first time on the earth we have created rich, scientific societies, and they are the most ugly and most unhappy. And in the past there was no scientific technology, no affluence, nothing of comfort, but humanity was existing in such a deep, peaceful milieu—happy, thankful. What has happened? We can be happier than anyone, but we have lost contact with existence.

And that existence is here and now, and an impatient mind cannot be in contact with it. Impatience is like a feverish, mad state of mind; you go on running. Even if the goal comes, you cannot stand there because the running has become just a habit.

Even if you reach the goal, you will miss it, you will pass by it because you cannot stop.

If you can stop, the goal need not be searched.

Zen Master Hui-Hai has said, "Seek, and you will lose; don't seek, and you can get it immediately. Stop and it is here. Run, it is nowhere."

Why do so many people on the path of yoga adopt an attitude of fight, struggle, overconcern with keeping strict rules, and warriorlike ways? Is this really necessary in order to be a yogi?

It is absolutely unnecessary—not only unnecessary, it creates all types of hindrances on the path of yoga. The warriorlike attitude is the greatest hindrance possible because there is no one to fight with. Inside, you are alone. If you start fighting, you are splitting yourself.

This is the greatest disease: to be divided, to become schizophrenic. And the whole struggle is useless because it is not going to lead anywhere. No one can win; on both the sides *you* are. So at the most, you can play; you can play a game of hide and seek. Sometimes part A wins, sometimes part B wins; again part A, again part B. In this way you can move. Sometimes that which you call good wins. But fighting with the bad, winning over the bad, the good part has become exhausted and the bad part has gathered energy. So sooner or later the bad part will come up. And this can go on infinitely.

But why does this warriorlike attitude happen? Why with most people does fighting start? The moment they think of transformation, they start fighting. Why? Because you know only one method of winning, and that is to fight.

In the outside world there is one way to be victorious, and

that is to fight—fight and destroy the other. This is the only way to be victorious in the outside world. You have lived in this outside world for millions and millions of years, and you have been fighting—sometimes getting defeated if you don't fight well, sometimes being victorious if you fight well. So it has become a built-in program to fight and be strong. There is only one way to be victorious, and that is through a hard fight.

When you move within, you carry the same program because you are acquainted only with this. And in the world within, just the reverse is the case: Fight and you will be defeated—because there is no one to fight with! In the inner world, let-go is the way to be victorious, surrender is the way to be victorious, allowing the inner nature to flow, not fighting, is the way to be victorious. Letting the river flow, not pushing it, is the way as far as the inner world is concerned. This is just the reverse.

But you are acquainted only with the outside world, so this is bound to happen in the beginning. Whoever moves within will carry the same weapons, the same attitudes, the same fighting, the same defenses.

Machiavelli is for the outside world. Lao Tzu, Patanjali, and Buddha are for the inside world. And they teach different things. Machiavelli says attack is the best defense: "Don't wait. Don't wait for the other to attack because then you are already on the losing side. You have already lost because the other has started. He has already gained, so it is always better to start. Don't wait to defend; always be the aggressor. Before somebody else attacks you, you attack him and fight with as much cunning as possible,

Machiavelli is for the outside world. Lao Tzu, Patanjali, and Buddha are for the inside world. And they teach different things.

with as much dishonesty as possible. Be dishonest, be cunning, and be aggressive. Deceive because that is the only way." These are the means that Machiavelli suggests. And Machiavelli is an honest man; that's why he suggests exactly whatsoever is needed.

But if you ask Lao Tzu, Patanjali, or Buddha, they are talking of a different type of victory—the inner victory. There, cunning won't do. Deceiving won't do, fighting won't do, aggression won't do—because whom are you going to deceive? Whom are you going to defeat? You alone are there.

In the outside world you are never alone. The others are there; they are the enemies. In the inside world you alone are there. There is no "other." There is no enemy, no friend. This is a totally new situation for you. You will carry the old weapons—but those old weapons will become the cause of your defeat.

When you change the world from without to within, leave all that you have learned from without. That is not going to help.

Somebody asked Ramana Maharshi, "What should I learn to become silent, to know myself?"

Ramana Maharshi is reported to have said, "For reaching the inner self, you need not learn anything. You need unlearning. Learning won't help—it helps you to move without. Unlearning will help."

Whatsoever you have learned, unlearn it, forget it, drop it. Move inside innocently, childlike—not with cunningness and cleverness but childlike trust and innocence. Not thinking in terms that someone is going to attack you—there is no one, so don't feel insecure and don't make any arrangements for your defense. Remain vulnerable, receptive, open.

That's what *shraddha,* trust, means. Doubt is needed outside because the other is there. He may be thinking to deceive you, so you have to doubt and be skeptical. Inside, no doubt, no skepticism, is needed. Nobody is there to deceive you. You can remain there just as you are.

That's why everybody carries this warriorlike attitude, but it is not needed. It is a hindrance—the greatest hindrance. Leave it outside. You can make it a point to remember that whatever is needed outside will become a hindrance inside. Whatsoever, I say unconditionally.

And just the reverse has to be tried. If doubt helps outside in scientific research, then faith will help inside in spiritual inquiry. If aggressiveness helps outside in the world of power, prestige, others, then nonaggressiveness will help inside. If a cunning, calculating mind helps outside, then an innocent, noncalculating, childlike mind will help inside.

Remember this: Whatsoever helps outside, just the reverse will do inside. So read Machiavelli's *The Prince*—that is the way to outside victory. And just reverse Machiavelli's *The Prince,* and you can reach inside. Just make Machiavelli stand upside down, and he becomes Lao Tzu—just in *shirshasan,* in the headstand. Machiavelli standing on his head becomes Patanjali. So read *The Prince;* it is beautiful—the clearest statement for the outside victory. And then read Lao Tzu's *Tao Te Ching* or Patanjali's *Yoga Sutras* or Buddha's *Dhammapada* or Jesus' *Sermon on the Mount.* They are just the contradictory, just the reverse, just the opposite.

Jesus says, "Blessed are the meek, for they shall inherit the earth"—meek, innocent, weak, not strong in any sense. "Blessed are the poor in spirit, for theirs is the kingdom of heaven." And Jesus makes it clear: "poor in spirit." They have nothing to claim; they cannot say, "I have this." They don't possess anything—knowledge, wealth, power, prestige. They don't possess anything; they are poor. They cannot claim, "This is mine."

We go on claiming, "This is mine, that is mine. The more I can claim, the more I feel I am." In the outside world, the greater the territory of your mind, the more you are. In the inner world, the lesser the territory of mind, the greater you are. And when the territory disappears completely and you have become a zero—then you are the greatest. Then you are the victorious. Then the victory has happened.

Warriorlike attitudes—struggle, fight, overconcern with strict rules, regulations, calculations, planning—this mind is carried inside because you have learned it, and you don't know anything else. You are almost blind to any other way. You cannot see it because eyes can see only what they have learned to see. If you are a tailor, then you don't look at faces, you look at clothes. Faces don't mean much; just by looking at the clothes you know what type of person is there. You know a language.

If you are a shoemaker, you need not even look at the clothes; the shoes will do. And a shoemaker can just look down on the street and know who is passing, just by looking at the shoe—whether he is a great leader, whether he is an artist, a Bohemian, a hippie, a rich man. Whether he is cultured, educated, uneducated, a villager—the shoemaker can know who he is just by looking at the shoe because the shoe gives all the indications. The shoemaker knows the language. If a man is winning in life, the shoe has a different shine. If he is defeated in life, the shoe is defeated. Then the shoe is sad, not cared for. And the shoemaker knows it. He need not look at your face. The shoe will tell him everything that he wants to know.

We learn everything, and then we become fixed in it. Then that's what we see. You have learned something, and you have wasted many lives in learning it. And it is now deeply rooted, imprinted. It has become part of your brain cells. So when you move within, there is simply darkness, nothing; you cannot see anything. The whole world that you know has disappeared.

It is as if you just know one language, and suddenly you are transported to a land where no one understands your language, and you cannot understand anybody's language. People are talking and chattering, and you feel simply that they are mad. It sounds like they are talking gibberish, and it seems very noisy because you cannot understand. They seem to be talking too loudly. If you can understand it, then the whole thing changes; you become part of it. Then it is not gibberish; it becomes meaningful.

When you enter within, you know only the language of the without. There is darkness within. Your eyes cannot see; your ears cannot hear; your hands cannot feel. Somebody needs to take your hand in his hand and move you onto this unknown path until you become acquainted, until you start feeling, until you become aware of some light, some meaning, some significance around you.

Once you have the first initiation, things will start happening. But the first initiation is a difficult thing because this is quite an about-face, a total about-face. Suddenly your world of meaning disappears. You are in a strange world. You don't understand anything—where to move, what to do, and what to make of this chaos. A master only means someone who knows. And this inside chaos is not chaos for him; it has become an order, a cosmos, and he can lead you into it.

Initiation means looking into the inner world through someone else's eyes. Without trust it is impossible because you won't allow your hand to be taken, you won't allow anybody to lead you into the unknown. And he cannot give you any guarantee.

No guarantee will be of any use. Whatsoever he says, you have to take it on trust.

In the old days, when Patanjali was writing his sutras, trust was very easy because in the outside world, too, particularly in the East and especially in India, they had created a pattern of initiation. For example, trades, professions belonged to families through heredity. A father would initiate the child into the profession, and a child naturally believes in his father. The father would take the child to the farm if he was a peasant and a farmer, and he would initiate him into his farming. Whatever trade, whatever business he was doing, he would initiate the child.

In the outside world in the East, everything was to be initiated—someone who knew the way would take you. This helped very much because you were acquainted with the process of initiation, of someone leading you. So when the time came for an inner initiation, you could trust.

And trust, *shraddha,* faith was easier in a world that was non-technological. A technological world needs cunning, calculation, mathematics, cleverness—not innocence. In a technological world, if you are innocent you will look foolish; if you are cunning you will look clever, intelligent.

Our universities are doing nothing but this: They make you clever, cunning, calculating. The more calculating, the more cunning you are, the more successful you will be in the world.

Quite the reverse was the case in the East in the past. If you were cunning, it was impossible for you to succeed even in the outside world. Only innocence was accepted. Technique was not valued too much, but the inner quality was valued very much.

In the past if a person was cunning and he made a better

shoe, nobody in the East would go to him. They would go to the person who was innocent. He might not make such great shoes, but they would go to the person who was innocent because a shoe is not just some *thing;* it carries the quality of the person who has made it. So if there was a cunning and clever technician, nobody would go to him. He would suffer; he would be a failure. But if he was a man of qualities, character, innocence, then people would go to him. Even if he made imperfect things, people would value his things more.

Kabir was a weaver, and he remained a weaver. Even when he attained enlightenment, he continued weaving. And he was so ecstatic that his weaving was not very good—he was singing and dancing and weaving! There were many mistakes and many errors, but his things were valued, highly valued.

Many people would wait for Kabir to bring something—it was not just a thing, a commodity; it was from Kabir! The very thing in itself had an intrinsic quality. It had come from Kabir's hands. Kabir had touched it. And Kabir was dancing around it while he was weaving it, and he was continuously remembering the divine, so the thing—the cloth or the dress or anything—had become sacred, holy. The quantity was not the question but the quality. The technical side was secondary; the human side was primary.

So even in the outside world in the East, they had managed a pattern so that when you turned inward, you would not be totally unacquainted with that world. Something you would know, some guidelines, some light would be in your hand. You would not be moving into total darkness. The whole society was moving around trust, faith, authentic sharing—then it was helpful. When one's time came to move within, all these things would help him to be initiated easily, to trust someone.

Fight, struggle, aggressiveness are hindrances. Don't carry them. When you move inward, leave them at the door. If you carry them, you will miss the inner temple; you will never reach it. With those things you cannot move inward.

As the modern man is in such a hurry, and Patanjali's methods seem to take so long, to whom are you addressing these lectures?

Yes, the modern man is in a hurry, and just the opposite will be helpful. If you are in a hurry, then Patanjali will be helpful because he is not in a hurry. He is the antidote. Your mind needs an antidote. Look at it this way: Because the western mind particularly—and now no other mind exists, only the western mind more or less everywhere, even in the East—is in a hurry, that's why it has become interested in Zen because Zen gives the promise of sudden enlightenment. Zen looks like instant coffee, and it has an appeal. But I know Zen won't help because the appeal is not because of Zen, the appeal is because of hurry. And then you don't understand Zen.

In the West, whatsoever is rumored about Zen is almost false; it fulfills a need of the mind that is in a hurry, but it is not true to Zen. If you go to Japan and ask Zen people, they wait for thirty years, forty years for the first *satori* to happen. Even for sudden enlightenment one has to work hard. The enlightenment is sudden, but the preparation is very long. It is just like when you boil water: You heat the water; then at a certain temperature—a hundred degrees Celsius—the water suddenly evaporates. Right—the evaporation is sudden, but you have to bring it up to a hundred degrees. The heating will take time, and heating depends on your intensity.

And if you are in a hurry, you don't have any heat because in a hurry you would have to have the Zen *satori,* or enlightenment, just by the way—if it can be attained, if it can be purchased. You would like to run and snatch it from somebody's hands. It cannot be done that way. There are flowers, seasonal flowers: You sow the seeds, and within three weeks the plants are getting ready—but within three months the plants have blossomed, gone, disappeared. If you are in a hurry, then it would be better to be interested in drugs than in meditation, yoga, Zen because drugs can give you dreams. Instant dreams—sometimes of hell, sometimes of heaven—then marijuana is better than meditation. If you are in a hurry, then nothing eternal can happen to you because the eternal needs eternal waiting. If you are asking for eternity to happen to you, you have to be ready for it. Hurry won't help.

There is a Zen saying: If you are in a hurry, you will never reach. You can even reach just by sitting, but in a hurry you can never reach. The very impatience is a barrier.

There is a Zen saying: If you are in a hurry, you will never reach. You can even reach just by sitting, but in a hurry you can never reach. The very impatience is a barrier.

If you are in a hurry, then Patanjali is the antidote. If you are not in any hurry, then Zen is also possible. This statement will look contradictory, but this is so. This is how reality is: contradictory. If you are in a hurry, then you will have to wait for many lives before enlightenment happens to you. If you are not in a hurry, then it can happen right now.

I will tell you one story that I like very much. It is one of the old Indian stories:

> Narada, a messenger between earth and heaven, a mythological figure, was going to heaven. He is just like a

postman; he goes up and down continuously, bringing messages from above, bringing messages from below. He continues his work. He was going to heaven, and he passed one very, very old monk sitting under a tree with his *mala,* his beads, chanting the name of Rama. The old man looked at Narada and said, "Where are you going? Are you going to heaven? Then do me a favor. Ask God how much more I have to wait"—even in the very question, the impatience is there—"and remind him also," said the old monk, "that for three lives I have been doing meditation and austerities. And everything that can be done, I have done; there is a limit to everything."

A demand, expectation, impatience . . .

Narada said, "I am going, and I will ask."

And just by the side of the old monk, under another tree, was a young man dancing and singing the name of God. Just as a joke, Narada asked the young man, "Would you also like me to ask about you, how much time it will take?"

But the young man was so much in his ecstasy that he didn't answer.

After a few days Narada came back. He told the old man, "I asked God, and he laughed and said, 'At least three lives more.' "

The old man threw down his *mala* and angrily said, "This is injustice! And whoever says God is just is wrong!"

Then Narada went to the young man, who was still dancing, and said, "Even though you have not asked, I asked on your behalf, but I am afraid to tell you now because that old man has got into such an angry state, he even would have hit me."

But the young man was still dancing, still not interested.

Narada told him, "I asked him, and God said to tell that young man that he should count the leaves of the tree under which he is dancing; the same number he will have to be born again before he attains."

The young man listened—and went into such ecstasy; he laughed and jumped and celebrated. He said, "So soon? Because the earth is full of trees, millions and millions. And just these leaves? The same number? So soon? God is infinite compassion, and I am not worthy of it!"

And it is said that immediately he attained. That very moment he became enlightened.

If you are in a hurry, it will take time. If you are not in a hurry, it is possible right this moment.

Patanjali is the antidote for those who are in a hurry, and Zen is for those who are not in a hurry. And just the opposite happens: People who are in a hurry become interested in Zen, and people who are not in any hurry become interested in Patanjali. This is wrong. If you are in a hurry, then Patanjali—because he will pull you down and bring you to your senses, and he will talk of a path so long, he will be a shock to you. And if you allow him to enter you, your hurry will disappear.

That's why I am talking; I am talking about Patanjali because of you. You are in a hurry, and I hope Patanjali will bring down your impatience; he will pull you down, back to the reality. He will bring you to your senses.

Many of the existentialist thinkers of the West—Sartre, Camus, and so on—have come to realize the frustration, hopelessness, and meaning-

lessness of life, but they have not known the ecstasy of a Patanjali. Why? What is missing? What would Patanjali have to say to the West at this point?

Yes, a few things are missing in the West that were not missing for Buddha in India. Buddha also reached to a point where Sartre is: the existentialist despair, the anguish, the feeling that all is futile, that life is meaningless. But when Buddha reached this point—feeling that everything is meaningless—there was an opening in India. It was not the end of the road. In fact, it was only the end of one road, but another opened immediately; the closing of one door but the opening of another.

That is the difference between a culture that is spiritual and a culture that is materialist. A materialist says, "This is all; there is nothing else to life." A materialist says that all that you can see is all that reality is. If that becomes meaningless, then there is no door open. A spiritual person says, "This is not all, the visible is not all, the tangible is not all." When the visible is finished, suddenly a new door opens and this is not the end. When it is finished, it is only a beginning to another dimension.

This is the only difference between a materialist conception of life and a spiritual conception of life—the difference of worldviews. Buddha was born into a spiritual world view. He also realized the meaninglessness of all that we do because death is there, and death will finish everything, so what is the point of doing or not doing? Whether you do or don't do, death comes and finishes everything. Whether you love or not, old age comes, and you become a ruin, a skeleton. Whether you live a poor life or a rich life, death annihilates both; it does not bother about who you are. You may have been a saint, you may have been a sinner—to death it makes no difference. Death is absolutely communist; it treats everybody equally. The saint and the sinner both fall down into the dust—dust unto dust. Buddha came to realize this, but the spiritual worldview was there; the milieu was different.

I have told this story of Buddha. He comes to see an old man, and he realizes that youth is just a passing phase, a momentary phenomenon. A wave in the ocean rising and falling, nothing of permanence in it, nothing of the eternal in it; just like a dream, a bubble ready to burst any moment. Then he sees a dead man being carried. In the West the story would have stopped here—with the old man, the dead man. But in the Indian story, after the dead man, he sees a *sannyasin*—that is the door. And then he asks his driver, "Who is this man, and why is he in ochre robes? What has happened to him? What type of man is he?"

The driver says, "This man has also realized that life leads to death, and he is in search of a life that is deathless."

This was the milieu: Life doesn't end with death. Buddha's story shows that after seeing death, when life feels meaningless, suddenly a new dimension arises. A new vision, *sannyas*—the effort to penetrate into the deeper mystery of life, to penetrate deeper into the visible to reach the invisible. To penetrate matter so deeply that matter disappears, and you come to the basic reality, the reality of spiritual energy, the *Brahma*.

With Sartre, Camus, Heidegger, the story ends with the dead man. The *sannyasin* is missing; that is the missing link.

In the West, materialism has become the worldview. Even so-called religious people in the West are all materialists. They may go to church, they may believe in Christianity, but that belief is not even skin deep. It is a social formality. One has to go to church on Sunday; it is the thing to do, the right

> Even so-called religious people in the West are all materialists. They may go to church, they may believe in Christianity, but that belief is not even skin deep. It is a social formality.

thing to do to remain "the right people" in the opinion of others. You are the right people doing the right things—a social formality. But inside, everybody has become a materialist.

The materialist worldview says that with death everything ends. If this is true, then there is no possibility of any transformation. And if everything ends with death, then there is no point in continuing to live. Then suicide is the right answer.

It is simply wonderful to see that Sartre went on living. He should have committed suicide a long time before his death because if he had really realized that life is meaningless, then what is the point? Either he had realized it or he was still hoping against it and had not realized it. What is the point of carrying the whole thing again and again every day, of getting up out of bed? If you have really felt that life is meaningless, how can you get out of bed the next morning? For what? To repeat the same old nonsense again? Meaningless. Why should you breathe at all?

This is my understanding: If you have truly realized that life is meaningless, breathing will stop immediately. What is the point? You will lose interest in breathing, you will not make any effort. But Sartre went on living and living and doing millions of things. The meaninglessness had not really penetrated very deeply. It is a philosophy, not yet a life. Not yet an intimate happening inside, just a philosophy. Otherwise, the East is open; why shouldn't Sartre come? The East says, "Yes, life is meaningless, but then a door opens." Then let him come to the East and try to find the door.

And it is not only that people have said it; for almost ten thousand years many have come to *realize* this point, and you cannot delude yourself about it. Buddha lived for forty years in ecstasy with not a single moment of misery. How can you pretend? How can you live a forty-year life acting as if you are ecstatic? And what is the point of acting? And not only one Buddha—thousands of buddhas are born in the East, and they have lived the most blissful of lives with not a single ripple of misery arising.

What Patanjali is saying is not a philosophy, it is a realized fact; it is an experience. Sartre is not courageous enough; otherwise there would be two alternatives: either commit suicide, be true to your philosophy, or seek a way to life, a new life. In both ways, you leave the old. That's why I insist that whenever a person comes to the point of suicide, only then does the door open. At that point, there are two alternatives: suicide or self-transformation.

Sartre is not courageous. He talks about courage, sincerity, authenticity, but is none of these. If you are authentic, then either commit suicide or seek a way out of the misery. If the misery is final and total, then why do you go on living? Be true to your philosophy. It seems that this despair, anguish, meaninglessness is also verbal, logical, but not existential.

It is my feeling that the existentialism of the West is not really existentialist; it is again a philosophy. To be existentialist means it must be a feeling, not a thinking. Sartre may have been a great thinker—he was—but he did not feel the thing, he did not live it. If you live despair, you are bound to come to a point where something has to be done, radically done, immediately done. A transformation becomes urgent, becomes your only concern.

You have also asked what is missing. The worldview, the spiritual worldview, is missing in the West. Otherwise, many buddhas could be born. The season is ripe—despair, meaninglessness is felt; it is in the air. The society has achieved affluence and found it lacking. Money is there, power is there, and man feels deep down totally impotent. The situation is ripe but the worldview is lacking.

The West needs the worldview of spirituality, so that those who have come to the end of their travels in this life should not feel that it is the end—a new door opens. Life is eternal. Many times you will feel that everything has ended, and suddenly something again starts. A worldview of spirituality is lacking. Once that worldview is there, many will start moving into it.

The trouble is that many so-called religious teachers from the East are moving to the West, and they are more materialist than you are. They are there simply for the money. They cannot give you the worldview of spirituality; they are salesmen. They have found the market because the season is ripe. People are hankering for something, not knowing what. People are finished with this so-called life, frustrated, ready to take a jump into something unknown, yet unlived. The market is ready for people to exploit, and there are many merchants from the East. They may be called *maharishis,* that makes no difference. Many merchants, salesmen, are moving to the West. They are just there for the money.

With a real master, you have to come to him—you have to seek him, you have to find him, you have to make efforts. A real master cannot go to the West because just by going, the whole point will be lost; the West has to come to him. And it will be easier for Western people to come to the East to learn the inner discipline, the awakening, and then go to the West and spread the new milieu. It will be easier for Western people to learn in the East, to be in the atmosphere of a spiritual master and then carry back the message—because you will not be a materialist if you go and spread the news in the West. You will not be a materialist because you have been materialistic enough; you are finished with it.

When poor people from the East go to the West, of course they start accumulating money. That's simple. The East is poor, and now the East is not hankering for spirituality, it is hankering for more money, more material gadgets, more engineering and atomic science. Even if a buddha were to be born, nobody would talk about him in the East. But India releases a small toy satellite, and the whole country goes mad and happy. What stupidity! A small atomic explosion, and India feels very happy and proud because she has become the fifth atomic power.

The East is poor, and the East is now thinking in terms of matter. A poor mind always thinks about matter and all that matter can give. The East is not in search of spirituality. The West is rich, and now the West is ready to seek.

I don't know what Patanjali would have said to the West. How can I know? Patanjali is Patanjali; I am not Patanjali. But this is what I would like to say: The West has come to a point where either suicide or a spiritual revolution will happen. These are the only two alternatives. I'm not saying this only about individual persons. This is so for the West as a whole. Either the West will commit suicide through atomic war, for which it is preparing, or there will be a spiritual awakening. And there is not very much time left. Within just a matter of years, the West will either commit suicide or will know the greatest spiritual awakening that has ever happened in the history of man. Much is at stake.

People come to me and they say, "You go on giving *sannyas*

without considering whether the person is worthy or not." I tell them that time is short, and I don't bother about it. If I give *sannyas* to fifty thousand people and only fifty prove to be true, that will be enough.

Within just a matter of years, the West will either commit suicide or will know the greatest spiritual awakening that has ever happened in the history of man. Much is at stake.

The West needs *sannyasins*. The story there has gone to the point where the dead man is being carried. Now a *sannyasin* has to appear in the West. And the *sannyasin* should be Western, not Eastern because the Eastern *sannyasin* will become a victim, sooner or later, of all that you can give to him. He will start selling; he will become a salesman because he comes from the starved East. Money is his god.

The *sannyasin* should be Western—one who comes from the roots of the West, who realizes the meaninglessness of life, who realizes the frustration of the whole effort toward materialism, who realizes the futility of all Marxism, communism, and all materialist philosophies. This frustration is in the blood of Western man now, in the very bones.

That's why my whole interest is to make as many Western people *sannyasins* as possible and send them back home. Many Sartres are waiting there. They have seen the death. They are waiting to see the ochre robe—and with the ochre robe, the ecstasy that follows.

Not to be identified with mind and body—I still don't know how to do it. I tell myself: You are not the mind, don't listen to your fear, love yourself, be content, etc., etc.

Please explain again how not to get identified, or, at least, why I still don't understand you.

It's not a question of telling yourself that you are not the mind, you are not the body because the one who is telling it is the mind. That way you are never going to get out of the mind. All telling is done by the mind itself, so you will be emphasizing the mind more and more. The mind is very subtle; you have to be very, very alert about it. Don't use it. If you use it, you strengthen it. You cannot use your mind to destroy your mind itself. You have to understand that this mind cannot be used for its own suicide.

When you say, "I am not the body," it is the mind saying so. When you say, "I am not the mind," it is again the mind saying so. Look into the fact; don't try to say anything. Language, verbalization is not needed. Just a deep look. Just look inside. Don't say anything. But I know your trouble. From the very beginning we are taught not to see but to say. The moment you see the rose you say, "How beautiful!" Finished. The rose is gone—you killed it. Now something has come between you and the rose. "How beautiful it is!"—these words now will function as a wall.

And one word leads to another, one thought to another. And they move in association; they never move alone. You will never find a single thought alone. They live in a herd; they are herd animals. So when once you have said, "How beautiful is the rose!" you are on the track; the train has started moving. Now the word "beauti-

> One word leads to another, one thought to another. And they move in association; they never move alone. They live in a herd; they are herd animals.

ful" will remind you of some woman you once loved. The rose is forgotten, the beautiful is forgotten, now comes the idea, a fantasy, imagination, memory of a woman. And then the woman will lead to many other things. The woman you loved had a beautiful dog. Here you go! And now there is no end to it.

Just see the mechanism of the mind, how it functions, and don't use the mechanism. Resist that temptation. It is a great temptation because you are trained for it. You work almost like a robot; it is automatic.

The new revolution that is coming into the world of education has a few proposals. One proposal is that small children should not be taught language first. First they should be allowed time to crystallize their vision, to crystallize their experiencing. For example, there is an elephant, and you say to the child, "The elephant is the biggest animal." You think you are not saying anything nonsensical, you think it is absolutely reasonable, and the child has to be told about the fact; but no facts need to be told. It has to be experienced. The moment you say, "The elephant is the biggest animal," you are bringing something that is not part of the elephant. Why do you say the animal is the biggest animal? Comparison has entered, which is not part of the fact.

An elephant is simply an elephant, neither big nor small. Of course, if you put it by the side of a horse, it is big, or by the side of an ant, it is very big; but you are bringing the ant in the moment you say the elephant is the biggest animal. You are bringing something that is not part of the fact. You are falsifying the fact; comparison has come in.

Just let the child see. Don't say anything. Let him feel. When you take the child to the garden, don't say the trees are green. Let the child feel, let the child absorb. Simple things, "The grass is green"—don't say it.

This is my observation, that many times when the grass is not green you go on seeing it as green—and there are a thousand and one shades of green. Don't say that the trees are green because then the child will see just green—any tree and he will see green. Green is not one color; it is a thousand and one shades.

Let the child feel, let the child absorb the uniqueness of each tree—in fact, of each leaf. Let him soak up, let him become like a sponge who soaks up reality, the facticity of it, the existential. And once he is well grounded and his experience is well rooted, then tell him the words; then they will not disturb him. Then they will not destroy his vision, his clarity. Then he will be able to use language without being distracted by it. Right now your language goes on distracting you.

So what is to be done? Start seeing things without naming them, without labeling them, without saying "good" or "bad," without dividing them. Just see and allow the fact to be there in your presence without any judgment, condemnation, appreciation whatsoever. Let it be there in its total nudeness. Be simply present to it. Learn more and more how not to use language. Unlearn the conditioning, the constant chattering inside.

This you cannot do suddenly. You will have to do it by and by, slowly. Only then, at the very end of it, can you simply watch your mind. No need to say, "I am not this mind." If you are not, then what is the point of saying it? You are not. If you are the mind, then what is the point of repeating that you are not the mind? Just by repeating it, it is not going to become a realization.

Watch, don't say anything. The mind is there like a constant traffic noise. Watch it. Sit by the side and see. See that this is mind. No need to create any antagonism. Just watch, and in watching, suddenly one day the consciousness takes a shift, changes, a radical change—suddenly from the object it starts focusing on the subject if you are a watcher. In that moment you know you are not the mind. It is not a question of saying; it is not a theory. In that moment you know—not because Patanjali says so, not because your reason, intellect, says so. For no reason at all, it is simply so. The facticity explodes on you; the truth reveals itself to you.

Then suddenly you are so far away from the mind, you will laugh at how you could believe in the first place that you were the mind, how you could believe that you were the body. It will look simply ridiculous. You will laugh at the whole stupidity of it.

"Not to be identified with mind and body—I still don't know how to do it." Who is asking this question, "How to do it?" See it immediately; who is asking this question, "How to do it?" It is the mind who wants to manipulate, it is the mind who wants to dominate. Now the mind wants to use even Patanjali. Now the mind says, "Perfectly true. I have understood that you are not the mind"—and once you realize that you are not the mind, you will become a super mind. The greed arises in the mind; the mind says, "Good. I have to become a super mind."

The greed for the ultimate, for bliss, the greed to be in eternity, to be a god, has arisen in the mind. The mind says, "Now I cannot rest unless I have achieved this ultimate, what it is." The mind asks, "How to do it?"

Remember, the mind always asks how to do a thing. The "how" is a mind question. Because "how" means the technique. The "how" means, "Show me the way so I can dominate, manipulate. Give me the technique." The mind is the technician. "Just give me the technique, and I will be able to do it."

There is no technique of awareness. You have to be aware to be aware. There is no technique. What is the technique of love? You have to love to know what love is. What is the technique of swimming? You have to swim. Of course in the beginning your swimming is a little haphazard. By and by you learn . . . but you learn by swimming. There is no other way. If somebody asks you, "What is the technique of bicycling?"—and you do bicycle, you know how to ride on the cycle—but if somebody asks, you will have to shrug your shoulders. You will say, "Difficult to say." What is the technique? How do you balance yourself on two wheels? You must be doing something. You are doing something but not as a technique; rather, as a knack. A technique is that which can be taught, and a knack is that which has to be known. A technique is that which can be transformed into a teaching, and a knack is that which you can learn but cannot be taught. So learn by and by.

A technique is that which can be taught, and a knack is that which has to be known. A technique is that which can be transformed into a teaching, and a knack is that which you can learn but cannot be taught.

And start from less complicated things. Don't suddenly jump to the very complicated. This is the last, the most complicated thing: to become aware of the mind, to see the mind and see that you are not the mind. To see so deeply that you are no longer the body and no longer the mind, that is the last thing. Don't jump. Start with small things.

You are feeling hungry. Just see the fact. Where is the hunger? In you, or somewhere outside you? Close your eyes, grope in your inner darkness, try to feel and touch and figure out where the hunger is.

You have a headache. Before you take aspirin, do a little meditation. It may be that aspirin is not needed then. Just close your eyes and feel where the headache is exactly, pinpoint it, focus on it. And you will be amazed that it is not such a big thing as you were imagining before, and it is not spread all over the head. It has a locus, and the closer you come to the locus, the more you become distant from it. The more diffused the headache, the more you are identified with it. The more clear, focused, defined, demarked, and localized, the more distant you are.

Then there comes a point where it is just like a needle tip: absolutely focused. Then you will come to have a few glimpses. Sometimes the needle tip will disappear; there will be no headache. You will be surprised, "Where has it gone?" Again it will come. Again focus; again it will disappear. At the perfect focusing, the headache disappears because at the perfect focusing, you are so far away from your head that you cannot feel the headache. Try it. Start with small things; don't jump to the last thing so immediately.

Patanjali also has traveled a long way to come to these sutras of *viveka*—discrimination, awareness. He has been talking about so many things as preparatory, as basic requisites, as very necessary. Unless you have fulfilled all that, it will be difficult for you just to nonidentify yourself with the mind and body.

So never ask "how" about it. It has nothing to do with "how." It is a simple understanding. If you understand me, in that very understanding you will be able to see the point. I don't say you will be able to understand it. I say you will be able to see it. Because the moment we say "understand," intellect comes in, the mind starts functioning. "Seeing it" is something that has nothing to do with the mind.

Sometimes you are walking on a lonely path, and the sun is setting, the darkness is descending, and suddenly you see a snake crossing the path. What do you do? Brood about it? Think about what to do, how to do it, whom to ask? You simply jump out of the way. That jumping is a seeing; it has nothing to do with mentation. It has nothing to do with thinking. You will think later on, but right now it is just a seeing. The very fact that the snake is there, the moment you become aware of the snake, you jump out of the way. It has to be so because mind takes time, and the snake won't take time. You have to jump without asking the mind. The mind is a process; snakes are faster than your mind. The snake will not wait, will not give you time to think what to do. Suddenly the mind is put aside, and you function out of the no-mind; you function out of your being. In deep dangers it always happens.

That is the reason why people are so attracted to danger. Moving in a speedy car, going one hundred miles per hour or even more, what is the thrill? The thrill is of no-mind. When you are driving a car one hundred miles per hour, there is no time to think. You have to act out of no-mind. If something happens, and you start thinking about it, you are lost. You have to act immediately; not a single moment is to be wasted. So the greater the speed of the car, the more and more the mind is put aside, and you feel a deep thrill—a great sensation of being alive as if you have been dead up to now and suddenly you have dropped all deadness and life has arisen in you.

Danger has a deep, hypnotic attraction, but the attraction is of no-mind. If you can do it sitting just by the side of a tree or a river or just in your room, there is no need to take such risk. It can be done anywhere. You have just to put the mind aside—wherever you can put the mind aside—and just see things without the mind interfering.

I have heard:

> An anthropologist in Java came across a little-known tribe with a strange funeral rite. When a man died, they buried him for sixty days and then dug him up. He was placed in a dark room on a cool slab, and twenty of the tribe's most beautiful maidens danced erotic dances entirely in the nude around the corpse for three hours.
>
> "Why do you do this?" the anthropologist asked the chief of the tribe.
>
> The chief replied, "If he does not get up we are sure he is dead!"

That may be the attraction of forbidden things. If sex is forbidden, it becomes attractive. Because all that is allowed becomes part of the mind. Try to understand this.

All that is allowed becomes part of the mind; it is already programmed. You are expected to love your wife or your husband; it is part of the mind. But the moment you start becoming interested in somebody else's wife, it is not part of the mind; it is not programmed. It gives you a certain freedom, certain freedom to move off the social track, where everything is convenient, where everything is comfortable—but everything is also dead. You become deeply interested in somebody else's woman. He may be fed up with that woman; he may be just trying to find out some other way to become alive again—he may even get interested in *your* wife.

The question is not of a particular woman or man. The

question is of the forbidden, the not allowed, the immoral, the repressed—that it is not part of your accepted mind. It has not been fed into your mind.

Unless a person is completely capable of becoming a no-mind, these attractions continue.

And this is the absurdity of the whole thing: that these attractions were created by the people who think themselves moral, puritans, religious. The more they reject something, the more attractive, the more inviting it becomes because it gives you a chance to get out of the rut; it gives you a chance to escape somewhere that is not social. Otherwise the society goes on and on, crowding you everywhere. Even when you are making love to your wife, the society stands there watching. Even in your privacy the society is there, as much as anywhere else, because the society is in your mind, in the program that it has given to your mind. From there it goes on functioning. It is a very cunning device.

Once in a while everybody feels the need just to do something that is not allowed, just to say yes to something for which they always have been forced to say no—just to go against oneself. Because that "oneself" is nothing but the program that the society has given to you.

The more strict a society, the greater possibility of rebels. The freer a society, the less possibility for rebels. I will call a society revolutionary where rebels disappear because they are no longer needed. I will call a society free when nothing is rejected, so there

I will call a society revolutionary where rebels disappear because they are no longer needed. I will call a society free when nothing is rejected, so there is no morbid attraction to it.

is no morbid attraction to it. If a society is against drugs, drugs will attract you—because they give you an opportunity to put the mind aside. You are burdened with it too much.

Remember, this can be done without being suicidal. The thrill that comes to you when you are doing something that the society does not allow is coming from a state of no-mind but at a very great cost. Just look at small children hiding somewhere behind a wall smoking. Watch their faces—they are so glad. They will be coughing, and tears will be coming to their eyes because taking smoke in and throwing it out is just foolish. I don't say it is a sin. Once you say it is a sin it becomes attractive. I simply say it is stupid, it is unintelligent. But watch a small child puffing a cigarette—watch his face. Maybe he is in deep trouble, his whole breathing system is feeling troubled, he is nauseated, tears are coming, and he is feeling tense—but he is still glad that he can do something that is not allowed. He can do something that is not part of his mind, which is not expected. He feels free.

This can be attained very easily through meditation. There is no need to move on such suicidal paths. If you can learn how to put the mind aside . . .

When you were born, you had no mind. You were born without any mind; that's why you cannot remember a few years of your life. The beginning years—three, four, five years—you don't remember them. Why? You were there; why don't you remember? The mind was not yet crystallized. You go backward; you can remember something that happened near the age of four, and then suddenly there is a blank, then you cannot go more deeply. What happened? You were there, very alive. In fact, more alive than you will ever be again because scientists say that at the age of four a child has learned, known, seen 75 percent of all the knowledge that is going to be there in his whole life. Seventy-five percent of the age of four! You have lived 75 percent of your life already, but no memory? Because the mind was not yet crystallized. The language was yet to be learned; things were yet to be categorized, labeled. Unless you can label a thing, you cannot remember it. How to remember it? You cannot file it in your mind somewhere. You don't have a name for it. So first the name has to be learned; then you can remember.

A child comes without mind. Why am I insisting on this? To tell you that your being can exist without the mind; there is no necessity for the mind to be there. It is just a structure that is useful in society, but don't get too fixated with the structure. Remain loose so that you can slip out of it. It is difficult, but if you start doing it, by and by you will be able to.

When you are going home from the office, on the way try to drop the office completely. Remember again and again that you are going home—no need to carry the office there. Try not to remember the office. If you catch yourself red-handed remembering something of the office again, drop it immediately. Get out of it, slip out of it. Make it a point that at home, you will be at home. And in the office forget all about the home, the wife, the children, and everything. By and by learn to use the mind and not to be used by it.

You go to sleep, and the mind continues. Again and again you say, "Stop!" But it doesn't listen because you have never trained it to listen to you. Otherwise the moment you say, "Stop!" it has to stop. It is a mechanism. The mechanism cannot say, "No!" You turn a fan on, it has to function; you turn it off, it has to stop. When you stop a fan, the fan cannot say, "No! I would like to continue a little longer."

It is a biocomputer, your mind. It is a very subtle mechanism, very useful; a very good slave but a very bad master.

So just be more alert; try to see things more. Live a few moments every day, or a few hours if you can manage, without the mind. Sometimes swimming in a river, when you put your clothes on the bank, then and there put the mind there also. In fact, make a gesture of also putting the mind there, and go into the river alert, radiant with alertness, remembering continuously. But I am not saying to verbalize; I am not saying that you go on saying to yourself, "No, I am not the mind" because then this is the mind. Just a nonverbal, tacit understanding.

Sitting in your garden, lying down on the lawn, forget the mind. There is no need. Playing with your children, forget the mind. There is no need. Loving your wife, forget the mind. There is no need. Eating your food, what is the point of carrying the mind? Or taking a shower—what is the point of taking the mind into the bathroom?

Just by and by, slowly . . . and don't try to overdo it because then you will be a failure. If you try to overdo it, it will be difficult, and you will say, "It is impossible." No, try it in bits.

Let me tell you one anecdote:

> Cohen had three daughters and was desperately looking around for sons-in-law. One such young man came on the horizon, and Cohen grabbed him. The three daughters were paraded in front of him after a lavish meal. There was Rachel, the eldest, who was decidedly plain—in fact, she was downright ugly. The second daughter, Esther, was not really bad looking but was decidedly plump—in fact, she

was fat. The third, Sonia, was a gorgeous, lovely beauty by any standard.

Cohen pulled the young man aside and said, "Well, what do you think of them? I have got dowries for them—do not worry. Five hundred pounds for Rachel, two hundred fifty pounds for Esther, and three thousand pounds for Sonia."

The young man was dumbfounded: "But why? Why do you have so much more dowry for the most beautiful one?"

Cohen explained, "Well, it is like this. She is just a teeny-weeny itsy-bitsy little bit pregnant."

So every day start getting a little bit pregnant—with awareness. Don't just become pregnant in a wholesale way. A little bit, by and by. Don't try to overdo it because that, too, is a trick of the mind. Whenever you see a point, the mind tries to overdo it, and of course you fail. When you fail, the mind says, "See, I was all the time saying to you this is impossible." Make very small targets. Move one foot at a time, even inch by inch. There is no hurry. Life is eternal.

But this is a trick of the mind. The mind says, "Now you have seen the point. Do it immediately—become nonidentified with the mind." And of course the mind laughs at your foolishness. For lives together you have been training the mind, training yourself, getting identified. Then in the sudden flash of a moment you want to get out of it. It is not so easy. Bit by bit, inch by inch, slowly, feeling your way, move. And don't ask too much; otherwise you will lose all confidence in yourself. And once confidence is lost, the mind becomes a permanent master.

People try to do this many times. For thirty years a person has been smoking, and then suddenly one day, in a crazy moment, he decides not to smoke at all. For one hour, two hours he carries on—but a great desire arises, a tremendous desire arises. His whole being seems to be upset, in chaos. Then by and by he feels this is too much. All his work stops; he cannot work in the factory, he cannot work in the office. He is almost always clouded by the urge to smoke. It seems too disturbing—such a great cost. Then in another crazy moment he takes a cigarette out of the pocket, starts smoking, and feels relaxed; but he has done a very dangerous experiment.

In those three hours when he didn't smoke, he has learned one thing about himself: that he is impotent, that he cannot do anything, that he cannot follow a decision, that he has no will, that he is powerless. Once this settles, and this settles in everyone by and by . . . You try once with smoking, another time with dieting, and another time with something else, and again and again you fail. The failure becomes a permanent thing in you. By and by you start becoming a piece of driftwood; you say, "I cannot do anything." And if you feel you cannot do it, then who can do it?

But the whole foolishness arises because the mind tricked you. It told you to immediately do something for which a great training and discipline is needed—and then it made you feel impotent. If you are impotent, the mind becomes very potent. It is always in proportion: If you are potent, the mind becomes impotent. If you are potent, then the mind cannot be potent; if you are impotent, the mind becomes potent. It lives on your energy, it lives on your failure; it lives on your defeated self, your defeated will.

So never overdo things.

I have heard about one Chinese mystic, Mencius, a great disciple of Confucius:

A man came to him who was an opium user, and he said, "It is very, very impossible. I have tried every way, every method. Everything finally fails. I am a complete failure. Can you help me?"

Mencius tried to understand his whole story, listened to it, came to understand what had happened: He had been overdoing it. He gave the man a piece of chalk and told him, "Weigh your opium against this chalk, and whenever you weigh it, write 'one'; next time write 'two,' again write 'three,' and go on writing on the wall how many times you have used opium. And I will come after one month."

The man tried. Each time he used opium, he weighed it against the chalk, and the chalk was disappearing by and by, very slowly, because each time he had to write "one," then with the same chalk "two," "three." . . . It started disappearing. In the beginning it was almost invisible; each time the quantity was reduced, but in a very subtle way. After a month when Mencius went to see the man, the man laughed. He said, "You tricked me! And it is working. It is so invisible—I cannot feel the change, but the change is happening. Half the chalk has disappeared—and with half the chalk, half the opium has disappeared."

Mencius said to him, "If you want to reach the goal, never run. Go slowly."

One of the most famous sentences of Mencius is: "If you want to reach, never run." If you really want to reach, there is no need even to walk. If you really want to reach, you are already there. Go slow! If the world had listened to Mencius, Confucius, Lao Tzu, and Chuang Tzu, there would be a totally different world. If you were to ask them how to manage our Olympics, they would say, "Give the prize to the one who gets defeated first. Give the first prize to the one who is the slowest walker, not the fastest runner. Let there be a competition, but the prize goes to one who is the slowest."

If you move slowly in life, you will attain much—and with grace and grandeur and dignity. Don't be violent; life cannot be changed by any violence. Be artful. Buddha has a special word for it; he calls it *upaya,* "Be skillful." It is a complex phenomenon. Watch every step, and move very cautiously. You are moving in a very, very dangerous place, as if moving between two peaks on a tightrope, like a tightrope walker. Balance each moment, and don't try to run; otherwise failure is certain.

"Not to be identified with mind and body—I still don't know how to do it. I tell myself: You are not the mind, don't listen to your fear, love yourself, be content . . ."

Stop all this nonsense. Don't say anything to the mind because the sayer *is* the mind. Rather, be silent and listen. In silence there is no mind. In small gaps when there is no word there is no mind. Mind is absolutely linguistic, it is language. So start slipping into the gaps. Sometime just look—as if you are an idiot, not thinking just seeing. Sometimes go and watch people who are known as idiots. They are simply sitting there—looking but not looking at anything. Relaxed, perfectly relaxed; their face has a beauty. No tension, nothing to do, completely at ease, at home. Just watch them.

If you can sit for one hour like an idiot every day, you will attain.

Lao Tzu has said, "Everybody seems to be so clever except me. I look like an idiot." One of the most famous novelists, Fyodor Dostoyevsky, wrote in his diary that when he was young he had an epileptic fit, and after the fit, for the first time he could understand what reality is. Immediately after the fit everything became absolutely silent. Thoughts stopped. Others were trying to find medicine and the doctor, and he was so tremendously glad. The epileptic fit had given him a glimpse into no-mind.

You may be surprised to know that many epileptics have become mystics, and many mystics used to have epileptic seizures—even Ramakrishna. Ramakrishna would go into a fit. In India we don't call it a "fit," we call it *samadhi*. Indians are clever people. When one is going to name a thing, why not name it beautifully? If we call it "no-mind," it looks perfectly good. If I say, "Be an idiot," you feel disturbed, uneasy. If I say, "Become a no-mind," everything is OK. But it is exactly the same state.

The idiot is below mind, the meditator is above mind, but both are without any minds. I am not saying that the idiot is exactly the same but something similar. The idiot is not aware that he has a no-mind, and the person of no-mind is aware that he has a no-mind. A great difference but also a similarity. There is a certain similarity between mad people and the realized ones. In Sufism they are called "the mad ones"—the realized ones are known as the mad people. They are mad in a way. They have dropped out of the mind.

By and by, learn it slowly. Even if you can have a few seconds of this superb idiocy when you are not thinking anything, when you don't know who you are, when you don't know why you are, when you don't know anything at all and you are deep in a non-knowledge state—in deep ignorance, in the deep silence of the ignorance, in that silence the vision will start coming to you that you are not the body, you are not the mind. Not that you will verbalize it! It will be a fact, just as the sun is shining there. You need not say that there is the sun and the shine. As the birds are singing—there is no need to say that they are singing. You can just listen and be aware and know that they are singing without saying it.

Exactly the same way prepare yourself slowly, and one day you will realize that you are neither the body nor the mind—nor even the self, the soul. You are a tremendous emptiness, a nothingness—a no-thingness. You are—but with no boundary, with no limitation, with no demarcation, with no definition. In that utter silence one comes to the perfection, to the very peak of life, of existence.

ABOUT THE AUTHOR

Osho's teachings defy categorization, covering everything from the individual quest for meaning to the most urgent social and political issues facing society today. His books are not written, but transcribed from audio and video recordings of extemporaneous talks given to international audiences over a period of thirty-five years. Osho has been described by the *Sunday Times* in London as one of the "1000 Makers of the 20th Century" and by American author Tom Robbins as "the most dangerous man since Jesus Christ."

About his own work, Osho has said that he is helping to create the conditions for the birth of a new kind of human being. He has often characterized this new human being as "Zorba the Buddha"—capable both of enjoying the earthy pleasures of a Zorba the Greek and the silent serenity of a Gautam Buddha. Running like a thread through all aspects of Osho's work is a vision that encompasses both the timeless wisdom of the East and the highest potential of Western science and technology.

Osho is also known for his revolutionary contribution to the science of inner transformation, with an approach to meditation that acknowledges the accelerated pace of contemporary life. His unique "Active Meditations" are designed to release the accumulated stresses of body and mind, so that it is easier to experience the thought-free and relaxed state of meditation.

MEDITATION RESORT

Osho Meditation Resort

THE Osho Meditation Resort is a place where people can have a direct personal experience of a new way of living with more alertness, relaxation, and fun. Located about one hundred miles southeast of Mumbai in Pune, India, the resort offers a variety of programs to thousands of people who visit each year from more than one hundred countries around the world.

Originally developed as a summer retreat for Maharajas and wealthy British colonialists, Pune is now a thriving modern city that is home to a number of universities and high-tech industries. The Meditation Resort spreads over forty acres in a tree-lined suburb known as Koregaon Park. The resort campus provides accommodation for a limited number of guests, in a new 'Guesthouse,' and there is a plentiful variety of nearby hotels and private apartments available for stays of a few days up to several months.

All resort programs are based in the Osho vision of a qualitatively new kind of human being who is able to both participate creatively in everyday life and to relax into silence and meditation. Most programs take place in modern, air-conditioned facilities and include a variety of individual sessions, courses, and workshops covering everything from creative arts to holistic health treatments, personal transformation and therapy, esoteric sciences, the "Zen" approach to sports and recreation, relationship issues, and significant life transitions for men and women. Individual sessions and group workshops are offered throughout the year, alongside a full daily schedule of meditations. Outdoor cafes and restaurants within the resort grounds serve both traditional Indian fare and a choice of international dishes, all made with organically grown vegetables from the resort's own farm. The campus has its own private supply of safe, filtered water.

For More Information

www.osho.com

A comprehensive Web site in several languages that includes an on-line tour of the Meditation Resort and a calendar of its course offerings; a catalog of books and tapes, a list of Osho information centers worldwide; and selections from Osho's talks.

Osho International
New York
E-mail: oshointernational@oshointernational.com
www.osho.com/oshointernational

OTHER TITLES IN THIS SERIES

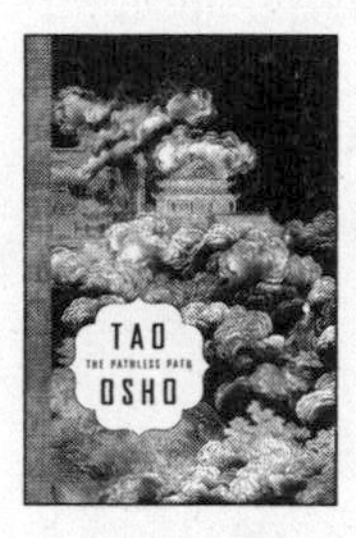

TAO: THE PATHLESS PATH

Contemporary interpretations of selected parables from the *Lieh Tzu* reveal how the timeless wisdom of this 2500-year-old Taoist classic contains priceless insights for living today.

ISBN: 1-58063-225-4 Paperback $11.95/$17.95 Can.

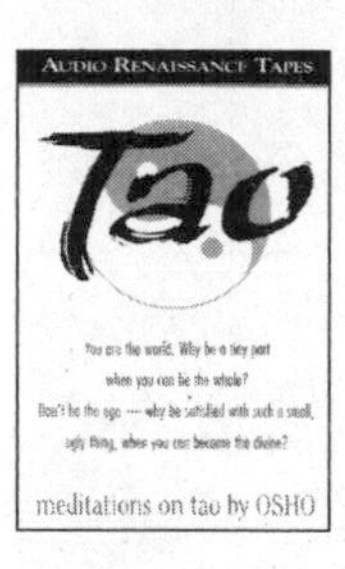

MEDITATIONS ON TAO

The audio book companion to *Tao: The Pathless Path* features verses from Ko Hsuan's *Classic of Purity* and from the *Tao Te Ching* of Lao Tzu.

ISBN: 1-55927-429-8 Audio Cassette $16.95/$23.50Can.

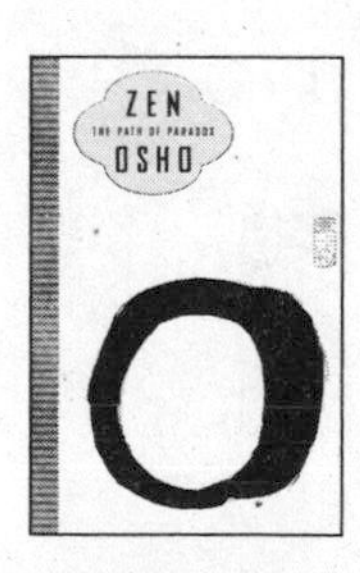

ZEN: THE PATH OF PARADOX

"Zen is not a philosophy, it is poetry. It does not propose, it simply persuades. It does not argue, it simply sings its own song. It is aesthetic to the very core." Osho calls Zen "the path of paradox" in this book, and unfolds the paradox through delightful Zen anecdotes and riddles.

ISBN: 1-58063-207-6 Paperback $14.95/$21.95 Can.

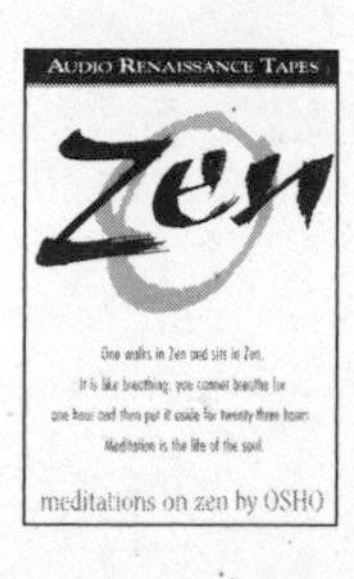

MEDITATIONS ON ZEN

Two classic Zen dialogues serve as a starting point for the journey into the world of Zen and how it can change every aspect of how we live our lives. By bringing our attention again and again to the here and now, we learn spontaneity and decisiveness, and to take life more playfully.

ISBN: 1-55927-428-X Audio Cassette $16.95/$23.50 Can.

OSHO AUDIOBOOKS

Recorded live in an open-air auditorium before an international audience, each Osho audiobook is not just a "lecture" but a profoundly relaxing meditation. The words are simple and direct, provoking an awareness of truths we have always known but perhaps have forgotten. The silences are profound, and are only deepened by the punctuations of birdsong or the whistle of a distant train. A treat for all the senses, and a quieting of the usual chatter of the mind.

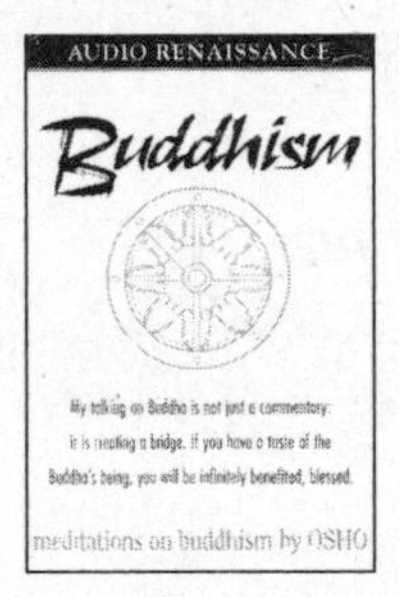

MEDITATIONS ON BUDDHISM
BY OSHO

ISBN: 1-55927-447-6
Audio Cassette
$16.95/$23.50 Can.

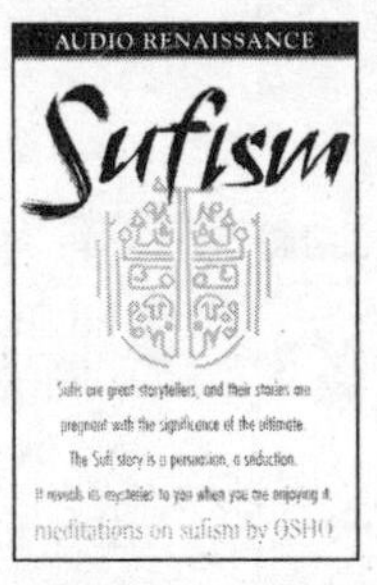

MEDITATIONS ON SUFISM
BY OSHO

ISBN: 1-55927-449-2
Audio Cassette
$16.95/$23.50 Can.

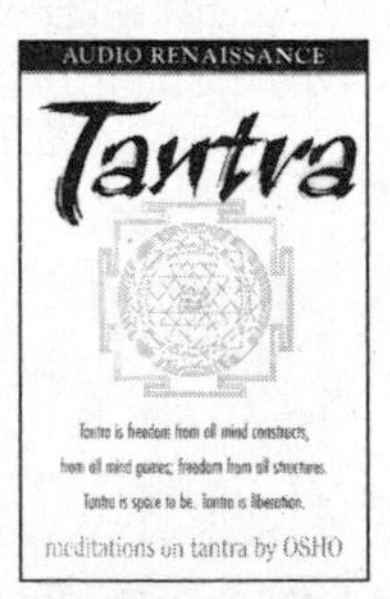

MEDITATIONS ON TANTRA
BY OSHO

ISBN: 1-55927-448-4
Audio Cassette
$16.95/$23.50 Can.

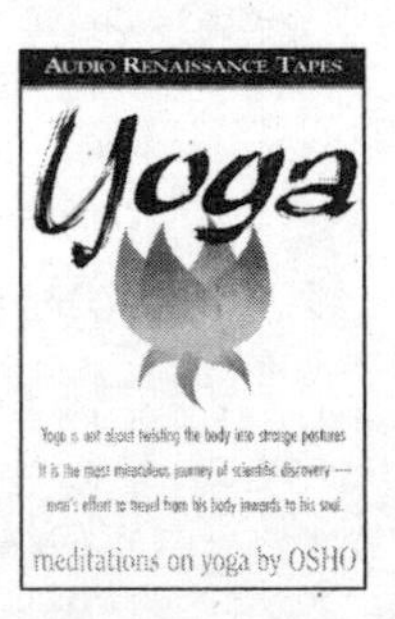

MEDITATIONS ON YOGA
BY OSHO

ISBN: 1-55927-430-1
Audio Cassette
$16.95/$23.50 Can.

FURTHER READINGS

SEX MATTERS

Sex matters to us all. The Osho approach to sex begins with an understanding of the importance of love in our lives, while acknowledging that the journey into love cannot exclude our innate biological energies. The tendency of religions, and society in general, to associate sex with sin is a great misfortune—Osho explains that sex is instead a unique door to self-discovery.

ISBN: 0-312-26160-8 Hardcover $25.95/$38.95 Can.

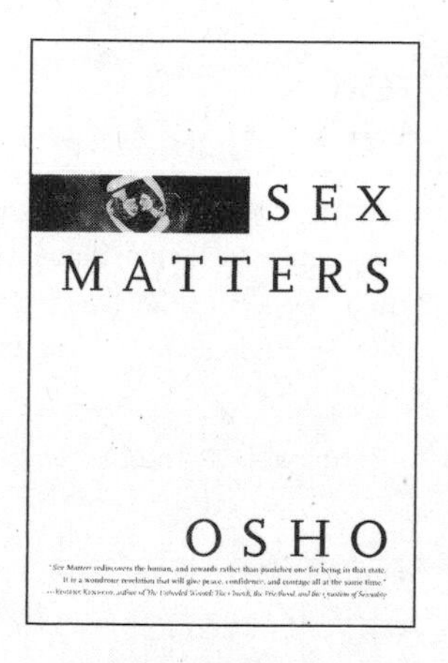

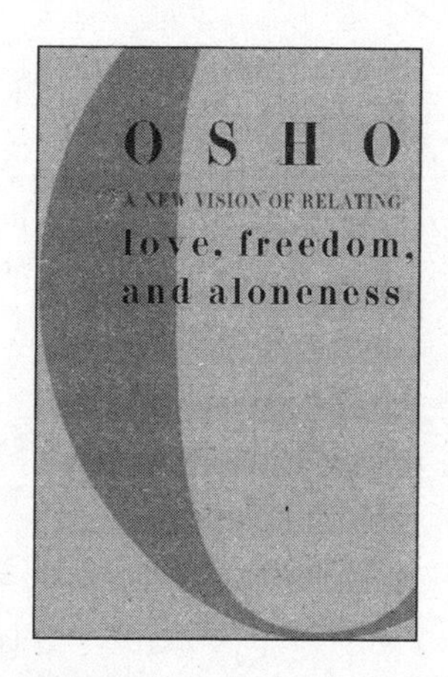

LOVE, FREEDOM, AND ALONENESS: A NEW VISION OF RELATING

This beautiful new book tackles the whole complexity of issues around relating—from sex to jealousy to compassion, from "falling in a ditch" to "rising in love." Whether you're just beginning a relationship or just ending one, or whether you're part of a happy couple or happy to be uncoupled and alone—reading these pages is like a heart-to-heart with a wise and perceptive friend.

ISBN: 0-312-29162-0 Paperback $14.95/$21.95 Can.

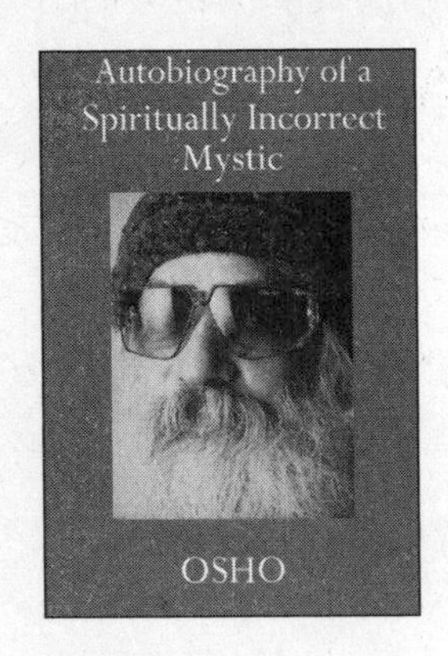

AUTOBIOGRAPHY OF A SPIRITUALLY INCORRECT MYSTIC

This delightful glimpse into the life of one of the most outrageous twentieth-century spiritual leaders answers some of the criticisms leveled at him for his seemingly outrageous behavior and his iconoclastic tendencies. He proves a fascinating man: a prolific writer and lecturer, highly educated, and deeply passionate about his own search for truth.

"[H]is autobiography is entertaining, insightful and for some, perhaps, even enlightening." – *Booklist*

Includes a 16-page black-&-white photo insert
ISBN 0-312-25457-1 Hardcover $25.95/$39.99 Can.

THE BOOK OF SECRETS: THE SCIENCE OF MEDITATION

Contemporary instructions and guidance for 112 meditation techniques, based on original sacred teachings from India. A unique and insightful overview of the entire science of meditation which allows individuals to find the method that suits them best.

ISBN: 0-312-18058-6 Hardcover $35.00/$46.99 Can.

THE BOOK OF SECRETS: KEYS TO LOVE AND MEDITATION

The audio companion to *The Book of Secrets*.

ISBN: 1-55927-486-7 Audio Cassette $16.95/$23.50

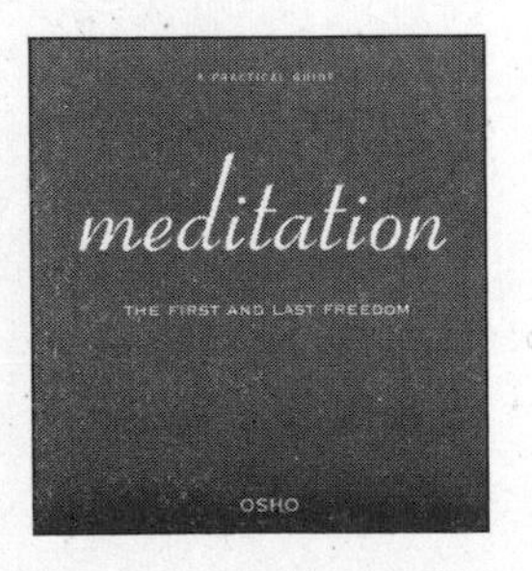

MEDITATION: THE FIRST AND LAST FREEDOM

A practical guide to integrating meditation into all aspects of daily life, which includes instructions for over 60 meditation techniques, including the revolutionary Osho Active Meditations™.

ISBN: 0-312-16927-2 Paperback $13.95/$17.99 Can.
ISBN: 0-312-14820-8 Hardcover $22.95/$35.99 Can.

SELF-DISCOVERY

THE INSIGHT SERIES: INSIGHTS FOR A NEW WAY OF LIVING

Osho's Insight Series aims to shine light on beliefs and attitudes that prevent individuals from being their true selves. With an artful mix of compassion and humor, Osho seduces his audience into confronting what they would most like to avoid, which in turn provides the key to true insight and power.

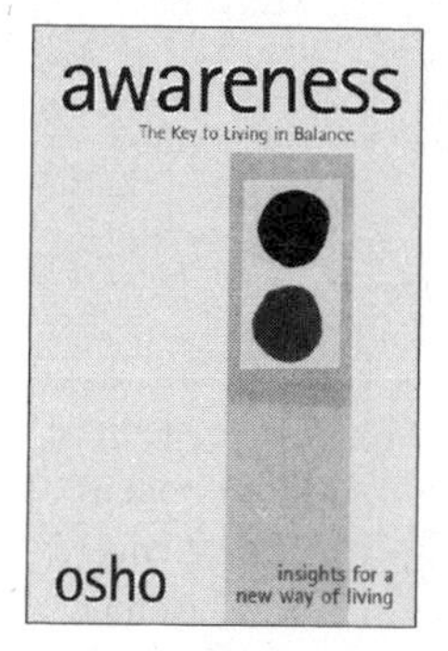

ISBN: 0-312-27563-3
Paperback
$11.95/$17.95 Can.

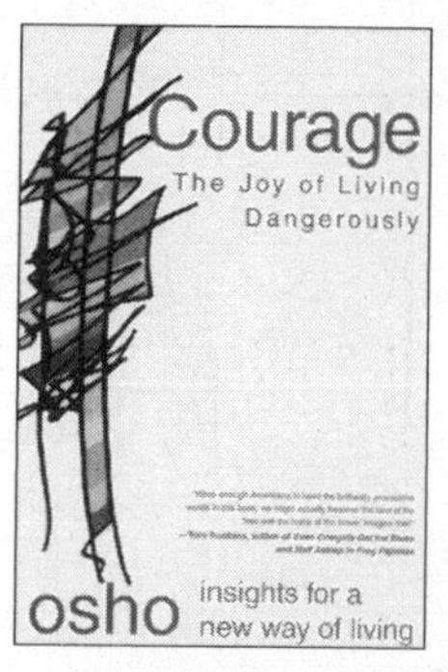

ISBN: 0-312-20517-1
Paperback
$11.95/$17.95 Can.

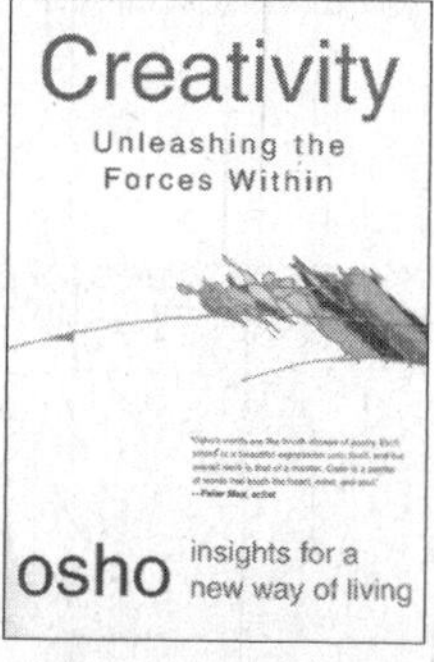

ISBN: 0-312-20519-8
Paperback
$11.95/$17.95 Can.

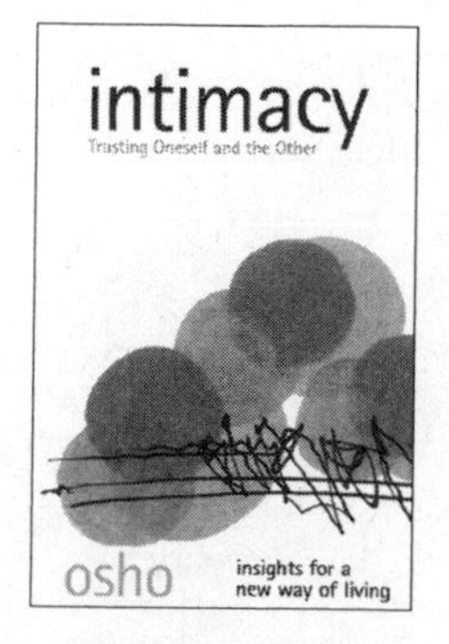

ISBN: 0-312-27566-8
Paperback
$11.95/$17.95 Can.

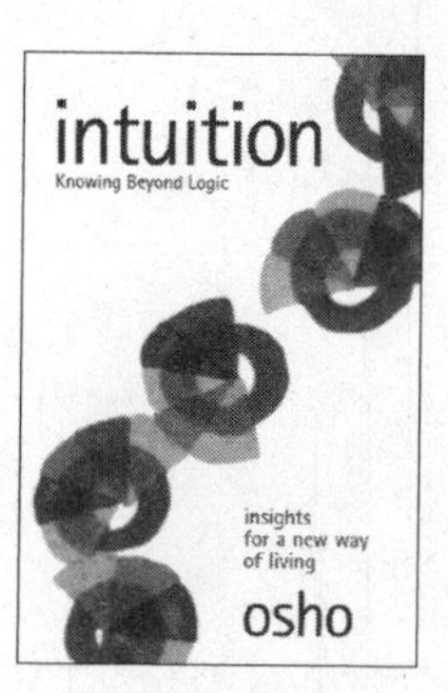

ISBN:0-312-27567-6
Paperback
$11.95/$17.95 Can.

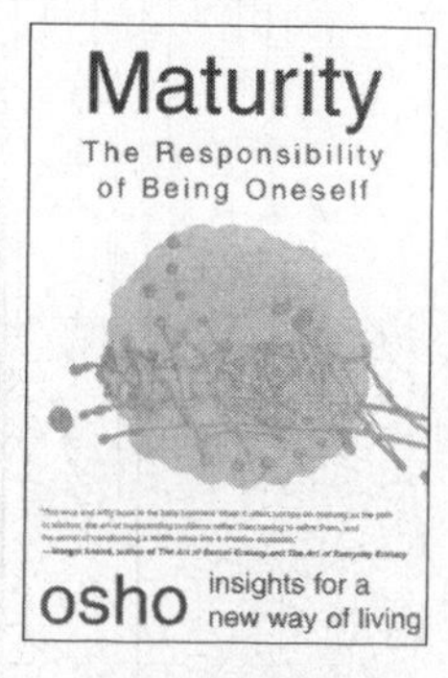

ISBN: 0-312-20561-9
Paperback
$11.95/$17.95 Can.